Water Culture in Roman Society

Ancient History

Volumes published in this Brill Research Perspectives title are listed at *brill.com/rpah*

Water Culture in Roman Society

By

Dylan Kelby Rogers

BRILL

LEIDEN | BOSTON

This paperback book edition is simultaneously published as issue 1.1 (2018) of *Ancient History*, DOI 10.1163/25425374-12340001.

Library of Congress Control Number: 2018936224

Typeface for the Latin, Greek, and Cyrillic scripts: "Brill". See and download: brill.com/brill-typeface.

ISBN 978-90-04-36894-1 (paperback)
ISBN 978-90-04-36897-2 (e-book)

This book is printed on acid-free paper and produced in a sustainable manner.

Dedicated to the Memory of Garrett G. Fagan (1963–2017),
Mentor, Friend, & Scholar of Roman Baths to All

Contents

Acknowledgements

This work is dedicated to the memory of Garrett Fagan, a scholar of Roman baths, whose work I have used extensively in my own research. But I have fond memories of an afternoon with Garrett in Rome in September 2015, while he was the Professor-in-Charge at the Intercollegiate Center for Classical Studies. I will never forget his warmth and joy, discussing various topics, from Roman baths to life in Rome.

I would like to thank Lee L. Brice, the editor of this series, in particular, for soliciting my current contribution, and for his steadfast guidance and patience along the way. Many scholars and friends have helped me refine my ideas and thoughts related to this work, especially Katherine Rinne and Tyler Jo Smith. Betsey Robinson, whether in Nashville or Athens, has always been extremely kind to discuss water with me. I wish to thank Dennis Kehoe for reading the section related to legal policies associated with water. Erika Jeck and her attention to detail improved the text immensely. I must thank the two anonymous readers, who both provided insightful and helpful comments. Further, discussions at various conferences have expanded my thinking on Roman water in general, particularly the meeting of the Frontinus Gesellschaft in Trier (May 2016), the October 2016 Summer Course at Kunsthistorisches Institut in Florence on "Wasser Formen," and the Idraulica Antica's November 2017 conference in Feltre, "Water and the Roman Cities and Settlements." Finally, the Blegen Library at the American School of Classical Studies at Athens, under the direction of Maria Tourna, provided the ideal workspace to complete this project. Any errors remain my own.

Editors' Note

We, the editorial board and Brill, are extremely pleased to launch *Ancient History*. We are confident that readers will find this journal useful and insightful as they navigate the active and ever-evolving field of ancient history.

The first issue of a new journal is an opportunity to present the scope and aims of the venture and to demonstrate where this publication fits into the vast array of resources already available to readers. After examining the resources currently on offer to readers working on, or interested in, the ancient world, including scholars, teachers, and students, we found there is both a need and a desire for publications which present extended discussions of historiography and the state of research on a range of topics in ancient Greek and Roman history. Surveys of topics in the field are occasionally published in professional journals, but recently these have tended to be limited in coverage and reach. Historiographic articles have also appeared inconsistently, except in the context of review articles, though these also are limited in scope, inconsistent in appearance, and dependent on publication trends. This pattern has resulted in gaps in readers' appreciation of recent work that has been completed and is in progress in a wide variety of subjects. This journal aims to help fill this gap.

Our intended audiences are diverse. While scholars obviously need access to such discussions to further their own research and catch up on recent work and trends, they are not the only constituency. Readers of various backgrounds, including students and general readers, seek discussions of recent works as part of their interest in the ancient world and the process of learning and exploring the field. Teachers seek to remain current in the field as they prepare class lessons, assignments, and lectures. As repositories of resources and laboratories of new research, libraries need access to scholarly articles on the state of research in any field as part of their mission and service.

The aim of *Ancient History*, therefore, is to present extended, peer-reviewed articles which offer commentary on the current state of research on an array of topics in ancient history. All articles are solicited from international scholars and discussions are long enough (c. 30–40,000 words) so that each author has an opportunity to present a comprehensive treatment of their topic, aiming to provide useful, up-to-date analysis and review for scholars, teachers, and students. Published both in print and on-line, issues will be updated periodically by authors to revitalize their commentary and analysis and to ensure citations remain up-to-date.

Focused on ancient history broadly understood, the journal has a broad scope in geographic and chronological terms—encompassing the Greek and Roman worlds, including the Mediterranean basin and Europe. Just as the Hellenistic and Roman Worlds expanded into Egypt and the Near East and then retracted, so does the geographic scope of the journal in accord with article topics. Chronologically, *Ancient History* seeks to cover topics from the Bronze Age to Late Antiquity. Topics and fields we will leave to other journals include ancient poetry in all forms, philosophy, and archaeology. The Ancient Near East and Egypt are generally outside our coverage, except when these regions fall within the history of the Hellenistic and Roman worlds.

In this first issue of the journal we have Dylan Rogers' treatment of Roman water culture. Studies of the relationship between water and Roman society have increased in number, detail, and popularity, especially over the last several decades. Whereas once only antiquarians investigated aqueduct routes, now scholars have brought more rigor and diverse approaches to studies of water culture, and it has even entered popular culture via the Internet and television. There is now such a variety of sub-topics, approaches, theories, and works (in multiple languages) that it is difficult for the non-specialist to keep track of it all. Rogers makes sense of the swirling currents of the field. He engages readers from the start by moving beyond the historiography to also present the various roles and relationships of water and Roman culture and the ways scholars have and are continuing to grapple with the topic. Water culture, as presented by Rogers, is revealed to be a complex and fascinating topic that has gone through, and continues to experience, a rapid evolution. Readers will find his article both useful and entertaining. We are pleased to be able to feature it as our premier contribution.

Water Culture in Roman Society

Dylan Kelby Rogers
American School of Classical Studies at Athens, Greece
dylan.rogers@ascsa.edu.gr

Abstract

Water played an important part of ancient Roman life, from providing necessary drinking water, supplying bath complexes, to flowing in large-scale public fountains. The Roman culture of water was seen throughout the Roman Empire, although it was certainly not monolithic and it could come in a variety of scales and forms, based on climatic and social conditions of different areas. This discussion seeks to define 'water culture' in Roman society by examining literary, epigraphic, and archaeological evidence, while understanding modern trends in scholarship related to the study of Roman water. The culture of water can be demonstrated through expressions of power, aesthetics, and spectacle. Further there was a shared experience of water in the empire that could be expressed through religion, landscape, and water's role in cultures of consumption and pleasure.

Keywords

water culture – Roman archaeology – aqueducts – baths – sanitation – fountains – spectacle – religion – identity – pleasure – landscape

1 Introduction

Water is transmutable and transformative. Human fascination with water often derives from the fact that water, governed by the laws of physics and other natural forces, changes form and state,[1] as well as transforms other entities by

1 Strang 2005, 98; Oestigaard 2011, 38.

 | DOI 10.1163/9789004368972_002

providing life and inflicting death, as a natural force in its own right.[2] Water is also part of an inherently shared, cross-cultural experience, as all humans must use it. Given the endless variety of ways in which humans interact with water on a daily basis, all waterforms (whether natural or artificially created) have the ability to link "social groups physically and topographically."[3] One needs to find clear and clean water for drinking and bathing. A person can experience a waterscape, or all of the natural water features of the environment, including rivers, lakes, springs, and seas, along with the various forms of precipitation, such as rain and snow—making water an integral part of one's interaction with the world.[4] Or one can find oneself in front of an artificial fountain, which displays water and demonstrates the power and grandeur of water that has been harnessed, even in the case of the smallest of water-displays. Regardless of an individual's encounter with water, there is always an associated *lived* experience with this vital and versatile element.

The Romans were fascinated and obsessed with water on a variety of levels. The term 'water culture' is used here in an attempt to bring together the various aspects and nuances of the relationship between water and Roman society. The idea behind water culture is not a novel one, and appears widely across modern scholarship. One of the first major studies on water culture in the ancient Greco-Roman world was Renate Tölle-Kastenbein's 1990, *Antike Wasserkultur*. Her monograph offers a general overview of water collection, distribution, and disposal, in addition to a discussion of water's use in notions of power and as an aesthetic element. Alain Malissard's 1994 monograph, *Les romains et l'eau*, explored water usage of the Romans, including utilitarian- and pleasure-related uses, engineering issues, and the notions of power associated with the control of water (specifically through aqueducts and the formal administration of water). In 1996, Maria Ricciardi and Valnea Santa Maria Scrinari published a volume documenting all of the elements of the hydraulic systems of Ostia, under the title, *La civiltà dell'acqua in Ostia Antica*. The authors, however, do not attempt to define the notion of a water civilization implied in the title. Betsey Robinson, in her 2001 PhD dissertation exploring the culture of water at Corinth, uses the term 'culture' over 'cult,' in order to widen her discussion of not only religious elements of water, but also social implications of water usage.[5] In Hennig Fahlbusch's 2008 edited volume on the water features of Hadrian's Villa, *Wasserkultur* is used as a broad term in

2 Chirassi Colombo 2004, 305; Strang 2005, 105. See especially Kamash (2008).
3 Strang 2005, 108.
4 Rogers 2013, 2, 6.
5 Robinson 2001, 14.

order to illustrate the impact of water on the villa itself, but the volume is only limited to the practical aspects of the water collection and distribution network there. Brian Campbell's 2012 monograph on rivers of the Roman world demonstrates how water impacted Roman culture at large, albeit he does not specifically discuss Roman water culture *per se*.[6] Wolfram Martini explores the *Wasserkultur* of Perge's fountain and gate system; yet again, this term is used to suggest the importance of water at the site, without offering much in terms of definitions.[7] This failing is also true of the recent conference volume *Fountains and Water Culture in Byzantium* (2016), the contents of which thoroughly investigate the role of water in Byzantium, but without formulating an explicit definition of water culture.

Recent scholarship in Roman studies has attempted to define elements of Roman culture. Scholars advocate reexamining modes of cultural influence, especially in the Roman period, moving away from charged terms, such as Hellenization and Romanization.[8] 'Culture' simply put is how a society's practices and beliefs differentiate it from another society.[9] The so-called 'cultural revolution' of the Romans, a phenomenon tied to their imperial project, is seen in "the conversion of wealth into social prestige that [allows for] new forms of culture [to] emerge."[10] Indeed, as will be demonstrated below, there was a fluid cultural exchange when it came to water in the Roman world. While Rome early on invested in water-related building projects, such as the construction of the Aqua Appia in 312 BCE, over time these projects became more refined and grew in scale and complexity. But even though elements of Roman water culture were adopted and implemented throughout the empire, there were still variations based on region and local social practices. Water culture, and perhaps Roman culture at large, should not be considered monolithic.

Water culture is a broad concept. First and foremost, because water is a naturally-occuring element employed by humans in innumerable artificial forms, water culture comprises the intersection of natural and artificial elements in society, the exchange between human and natural realms. Secondly, water culture is composed of the specific, and sometimes idiosyncratic, forms of water manipulation through which a society achieves seemingly limitless

6 For example, see his section on the appearance of rivers in Roman literature, religion, and art (2012, 118–59).

7 Martini 2016.

8 See Wallace-Hadrill (2008, 17–28) for a full discussion of these issues.

9 Wallace-Hadrill 2008, 28–9; Spawforth 2012, 4. See Wallace-Hadrill's discussion of 'culture' (2008, 28–32).

10 Wallace-Hadrill 2008, 37.

goals: hydration, agricultural irrigation, decoration, public and personal hygiene, hydraulic power, and so on. Finally, any given water culture will bear different social implications throughout all levels of a society. Water is omnipresent, and therefore, whether visible or invisible, impacts all aspects of culture writ large. Thus, water culture, defined simply yet succinctly, is the set of water-related practices that both express and shape a society's perception of its place within the natural order, in relation to foreign societies, and concerning its own constituent participants.

Romans had an expansive and diverse water culture, which stretched throughout the empire, linking all of the various inhabitants over time. In order to understand better the water culture of the Romans, the following discussion employs a wide body of evidence. First, ancient literary sources are presented to demonstrate Roman attitudes on water, especially in terms of the inherent positive and negative qualities of water. Second, ancient water administration and legal policies associated with water are presented to illustrate the ways in which Romans themselves distributed water in public and private contexts throughout the empire. Third, a variety of archaeological evidence is presented to show the ubiquity of water in the Roman world, including aqueducts, baths, sanitation, water-displays, and hydraulic power. Fourth, regional trends of water usage will be offered, in order to demonstrate that, while water was employed in all parts of the empire, it could be used in different ways, according to social and climatic reasons. Finally, Roman water culture will be explored more holistically, in efforts to understand the ways in which water permeated different aspects of Roman society. The modern scholarship on Roman water is extensive, yet the ensuing discussion is meant to illustrate the wide body of evidence (archaeological, literary, epigraphic, etc.) that is constantly changing and impacting conceptions of water in the Roman world. The approaches of different scholars, trained in different schools of thought across the world, come together here—demonstrating the complicated nature of Roman water culture.

2 Ancient Roman Sources on Water

Stemming from a long Greek tradition of observing the properties of water, such as that of the Presocratics, the Romans knew much about water and were able to tap into its resources in a variety of ways.[11] The Romans classified

11 For more on the Presocratics and their thoughts on water, first see Vitruvius (*De arch.* 8.*praef.*1) and Seneca (*QNat.* 3.22). See also the most recent edited volumes of Curd and

waters based on their inherent qualities, based on an understanding of what made 'good' and 'bad' waters. 'Good' water was in constant motion, had a good taste, and was healthy, while 'bad' water was usually construed as the opposite. Water was also transformative, whether its composition was changed because of its own environment, or it was able to transform its consumers in some way.

Four prose authors, Vitruvius, Seneca the Younger, Pliny the Elder, and Frontinus, provide useful Roman views on water, especially as these works are scientific or administrative in nature. Each of these authors explains the properties of water and offers insights on the element. Their thoughts seem to reflect a commonality of Roman attitudes towards water, demonstrating the extent to which Romans understood the properties of this vital resource and how to harness its power for utilitarian and restorative purposes. Other literary sources, especially poetry, are mentioned here only where relevant.[12]

Vitruvius is widely known for his treatise on architecture (*De architectura*), probably written between 30–20 BCE. The ten books of the work explore a variety of topics that would have been crucial for the Roman architect or engineer to understand, including the layout of cities (Book 1), building materials (Book 2), temples (Books 3 and 4), public buildings (Book 5), private buildings (Book 6), decorative details of structures (Book 7), water (Book 8), sundials and clocks (Book 9), and machines (Book 10).[13] Within Book 8, Vitruvius discusses the four elements (preface), finding water (chapter 1), rainwater (chapter 2), the nature of different waters (chapter 3), testing water (chapter 4), methods for leveling earth for water infrastructures (chapter 5), and aqueducts and piping (chapter 6). Chapter 3's discussion of waters presents hot waters (1–5), poisonous waters (15–18), intoxicating waters (20), and springs that can harm (21–23). By demonstrating the properties of these different waters, Vitruvius ensures that subsequent architects and engineers know which types of waters are the best to collect. Scholars have shown that Vitruvius was relying on Greek sources for Book 8, especially from Hellenistic Pergamon.[14] If this is indeed the case, that means Vitruvius' discussion, while based in truth, might

Graham (2008). All translations of ancient texts are taken from the Loeb Classical Library, unless otherwise noted.

12 See Rogers (2015, 80–129) for a longer discussion of literary sources related to Romans' perceptions of water.

13 Rowland and Howe (1999, 1–18) provide a succinct introduction to Vitruvius and his treatise. For more on the notion of the Roman 'architect,' see Anderson (2014), who discusses all known Roman architects.

14 Lewis 1999; Wilson 2008, 298–99.

not actually reflect the state of Roman aqueduct technologies at the end of the first century BCE.

Seneca the Younger composed one of the first Roman treatises on scientific matters, the *Naturales Quaestiones*, in the early 60s CE. The seven books of the work deal with a variety of issues related to meteorology, including celestial phenomena (e.g., meteors, comets, thunder, lightning), terrestrial waters, precipitation, winds, earthquakes, and the sources of the Nile.[15] Seneca, a Stoic, presents in the *Natural Questions* an in-depth physical description of the various meteorological phenomena, in order to understand the nature of the benevolent, caring god, who sends signs through phenomena. Book 3 discusses terrestrial waters, including how water impacts health (3.2.1–2), movement of water and its relation to topography (3.3.1), rivers (3.4–19), varieties of water (3.20), deadly waters (3.21) and deadly waters without bad tastes or smells (3.25), stoicism and eternal waters (3.22), and hot waters (3.24).[16]

In Seneca's discussion of the nature of water, there is a passage of particular importance for understanding water in Roman thought:

> Aut stant omnes aquae aut eunt aut colliguntur aut uarias habent uenas. Aliae dulces sunt, aliae uarie asperae; quippe interueniunt salsae amaraeque aut medicatae, ex quibus sulphuratas dicimus, ferratas, aluminosas: indicat uim sapor. Habent praeterea multa discrimina, primum tactus: frigidae calidaeque sunt; deinde ponderis: leues et graues sunt; deinde coloris: purae sunt, turbidae, caeruleae, luridae, deinde salubritatis: sunt enim utiles, sunt mortiferae, sunt quae cogantur in lapidem, quaedam tenues, quaedam pingues; quaedam alunt, quaedam sine ulla bibentis ope transeunt, quaedam haustae fecunditatem afferunt.
>
> SEN. *QNAT.* 3.2.1–2

> All waters are still, or running, or collected, or occupy various subterranean channels. Some are sweet, others have flavors that are disagreeable in different ways; among them are the salty, the bitter, and the medicinal. In the last category I mean sulphur, iron, and alum waters. The taste indicates the properties. They have many other distinctive qualities in addition. First, there is touch: they are hot or cold. Then weight: they are light or heavy. Then color: they are clear, muddy, blue, yellowish. Then their

15 For more on the *Natural Questions*, see: Gross (1989), Gauly (2004), Hine (2010), and Williams (2012). Hine (2010) and Williams (2012) have reorganized the order of the books, placing Book 3, on terrestrial waters, at the beginning of the sequence.

16 For more on Book 3, see Gross (1989, 103–47), Gauly (2004, 96–104), and Berno (2012).

> effect on health: for some are wholesome, others are deadly. There are certain waters which thicken into rock, others are thin or fat. Some give nourishment, some pass through without any benefit to the drinker; and some waters, when drunk stimulate fecundity.
>
> TRANS. T.H. CORCORAN

This succinct passage encapsulates the Roman psyche regarding waters' inherent qualities, which framed how the Romans interacted with water in their daily lives. Of special note is the way in which Seneca discusses the transformative properties of water, giving life or bringing death, based on its composition.[17] Thus, water has the ability to nourish humans, but it also has the ability to transform and alter in a negative direction.

Pliny the Elder, in Book 31 of his *Historia Naturalis*, explores natural phenomena, in a similar vein to Seneca.[18] Pliny describes a great deal about water: medicinal properties of water (31.1), waters and their qualities (31.2), classes of water, including healing and curative (31.3–17), marvels associated with water (31.18), deadly waters (31.19), beneficial waters (31.21), water finding techniques (31.26–28), varieties of water (31.29), phenomena of waters (31.30), water pipes (31.31), hot and medicinal springs (31.32), medicinal uses of sea water (31.33–37), salt (31.39–45), soda (31.46), and sponges (31.47).

Finally, the commentary, *De aquaeductu urbis Romae*, of the year 98 CE by Sextus Iulius Frontinus, provides important insight into the construction and management of the city of Rome's water infrastructure.[19] Frontinus was installed the *curator* of the *cura aquarum* under Nerva in 97 and then flourished under Trajan, so he had an intimate knowledge of the water supply of the city of Rome.[20] While much of the work is technical or legal (e.g., distribution capacity of aqueducts or the legal rights of water servitudes), Frontinus provides glimpses into the nature of water, through his descriptions of certain aqueducts. The water of the Aqua Marcia was known for having a greenish

---

17 For more on the taste of water and its transformation of other elements, see Sen. *QNat.* 3.20.1–2.

18 The bibliography on Pliny the Elder is immense, but Healy (1999) offers an important discussion on science in the *Natural History*, and Gibson and Morello (2011) offers a wide array of essays on Pliny.

19 For more on Frontinus in general, see: Evans (1997); Bruun (2003); Peachin (2004). The most recent editions of Frontinus are Del Chicca (2004, in Italian), Rodgers (2004), whose introduction (1–20) offers a succinct understanding of the author and work, and Paniagua (2016, in Spanish).

20 See below, 11–13, for a full discussion of the *cura aquarum*.

color (7.1).[21] The Aqua Alsietina/Augusta was known for having no redeeming or consumable qualities for humans, so it was delivered to the Transtiberium for use in Augustus' Naumachia (11.1).[22] But Frontinus also indicates that the aqueduct supplied water to some farms and gardens in the area, in addition to acting as an emergency water source for fountains across the river (11.1–2). The Anio Novus had water that could sometimes turn a muddy color, because the banks of the river were loose (15.1–2).

These four authors share a few salient points of interest. First, the importance of the classification of water is present throughout. Seneca divides water not only into celestial or terrestrial (*QNat.* 3.23), but also by properties that can then give water its own specific tastes, medicinal properties, odors, and temperatures (*QNat.* 3.20.2). And just as there are a number of different liquids in nature, so too can there be a variety of waters to classify (Vitr. *De arch.* 8.3.26).

Furthermore, other literary texts mention that beneficial waters must be moving.[23] Pliny the Elder reports that physicians know that running water is better for those who drink it, due to the agitation of the currents in the water, than stagnant waters (*stagnantes*).[24] Because the water's impurities are removed through its motion, it can be used without concern for one's health. In fact, the importance of moving water extends well beyond its potability. The waters used in purifying rituals in Roman religious practice must also be moving.[25] Thus, in various aspects of Roman life, the importance of moving water, over stagnant, was stressed.

These authors also emphasize the transformative nature of water, both in terms of water's ability to alter its human consumers and water's own changeable status. Just as wine can take on the properties of the environment in which its grapes are cultivated, so, too, can water take on the quality of the soils that it passes through (Vitr. *De arch.* 8.3.4, 8.3.12). Seneca explores the ways in which the taste of water can be affected by its environment:

---

21 Frontinus curiously does not include any discussion of the pleasant drinking nature or coolness of the waters of the Aqua Marcia, as Vitruvius (*De arch.* 8.3.1) or Pliny (*HN* 31.24) do.

22 See also *Res Gestae* (22.4); Taylor (2000, 169–200), who describes of the aqueduct, along with the location of the *Naumachia* of Augustus.

23 Verg. *G* 4.25; Ov. *Fast.* 5.210; Stat. *Silv.* 1.3.17–18; Hor. *Epod.* 1.14.29.

24 Plin. *HN* 31.21.

25 Liv. 1.45.6–7; Ov. *Fast.* 4.778; Ov. *Met.* 3.27; Columella *Rust.* 12.4.3; Tac. *Hist.* 4.53; Valerius Flaccus 4.420–423; Sil. 8.125; Festus 152.11–13 L. On the necessity for moving water for religious use, see *Thesaurus cultus et rituum antiquorum* [*ThesCRA*] 2.3a.IV.A (s.v., Purificazione, Romana, Mezzi impiegati nelle purificazioni, liquidi e unguenti; V. Saladino).

> At quare aquis sapor uarius? Propter quattuor causas: ex solo prima est, per quod fertur; secunda ex eodem, si mutatione eius nascitur; tertia ex spiritu, qui in aquam transfiguratus est; quarta ex uitio, quod saepe concipiunt corruptae per iniuriam. Hae causae saporem dant aquis uarium, hae medicatam potentiam, hae grauera spiritum odoremque pestiferum, hae leuitatem grauitatemque, <hae> aut calorem aut nimium rigorem. Interest utrum loca sulphure an nitro an bitumine plena transierint; hac ratione corruptae cum uitae periculo bibuntur.
>
> SEN. *QNAT.* 3.20.1–2

> But why the variety of taste in water? There are four causes. The first is from the soil through which the water is carried; the second also depends on the soil if the water is produced by a transmutation of earth into water; the third comes from the air which was transformed into water; the fourth from a pollution which water often receives when it has been corrupted by harmful substances. These causes give water its different taste, its medicinal power, its disagreeable exhalation and pestilential odor, as well as its unwholesomeness, heat or excessive cold. It makes a difference whether it passes through places full of sulphur, nitre, or bitumen. When water is polluted this way it is a risk of life to drink it.
>
> TRANS. T.H. CORCORAN

Seneca cites a variety of ways in which water is malleable. For example, water might be transformed by interacting with earth and air (an idea possibly rooted in the conceptualization of the canonical four elements). Contact with different elements can change water itself, such as in taste, odor, and wholesomeness. When water's healthful qualities are jeopardized, then it has the power to harm those who drink it. Therefore, these ancient sources also report that water can adversely affect people, potentially causing death, intoxication, forgetfulness, dullness, or tooth loss.[26] In order to choose the healthiest and best tasting water, one must always be aware of water sources.

---

26 For deadly waters, see: Vitr. *De arch.* 8.3.21–23; Sen. *QNat.* 3.2.1–2, 3.21, 3.25; Plin. *HN* 31.19. Poisonous waters can be found in Vitruvius (*De arch.* 8.3.15–20), with intoxicating waters in the same section (8.3.20). There are two polar opposite springs near the river Hercynnus in Boeotia: one induces forgetfulness and the other causes rememberance (Plin. *HN* 31.11). Men becoming dull from water is found in Vitruvius (*De arch.* 8.22) and Pliny (*HN* 31.12). For tooth loss, see Vitruvius (*De arch.* 8.3.23). Pliny, however, reminds the reader that there are plenty of healing qualities from a variety of waters (*HN* 31.3–12).

Roman authors also stress the necessity of water. On a superficial level, Pliny the Younger mentions that water is necessary for the upkeep of a villa (*Ep.* 2.17.25). Of course, water is crucial not only for drinking, but also for a variety of other utilitarian uses, as Vitruvius reminds his readers (*De arch.* 8.*praef.*3). Water is used for raising animals and various foodstuffs (Vitr. *De arch.* 8.3.28). Columella warns his reader to water plants thoroughly, lest they die (*Rust.* 10.143–44). Thus, the harnessing of water by the Romans is the catalyst for the flourishing of all forms of life, not only of humans, but also of flora and fauna necessary for survival.

3 Roman Water Management: Administration, Distribution and Legal Regulations

Roman communities tended to ensure that inhabitants of the empire had access to water, whether through public or private means. Although Roman water management remains a complicated and ever-changing subject to modern scholars, given the wide array of available evidence spanning the entire empire and several centuries, the administration, distribution, and legal regulations of water provide insight into the types of access Romans may have had to this necessary life-giving element. This section discusses the ways that Romans made water accessible to a variety of constituencies, while highlighting modern debates in Roman water management. There were a number of administrative and legal mechanisms for the control of water on a variety of levels, which evidences the importance of water in their culture at large. That being said, vast differences in water management programs (e.g., public, private, planned, or ad hoc) found across the Roman world demonstrate the overall locally autonomous nature of water systems throughout the empire.

Before turning to the actual administration, distribution, and legal regulation of water, a brief note should be made about types of water and some flood management strategies. The Romans distinguished between public and private water sources. Private water sources might include wells, springs, and streams, while public water typically comprised rivers, seas, and aqueducts.[27] These notions of public and private water sources will guide the ensuing discussion of how a Roman could access water.

Of these various public water sources, rivers especially required close administrative attention. Rivers had to be controlled (to prevent potential

27 Bannon 2009, 13.

destruction) and monitored (particularly in terms of economic interests).[28] The Tiber River was (and still is) prone to flooding.[29] For example, the flooding Tiber ruined the 13 BCE inauguration of Lucius Cornelius Balbus' theater in the Campus Martius when its overflowing waters submerged part of the theater itself.[30] In order to facilitate the control of rivers, then, flood management strategies were put into place, and aediles might have originally maintained the Tiber River and its banks. By the Julio-Claudian period, however, an office had been established, perhaps with five officers, the *curatores riparum et alvei Tiberis* (curators of the banks and the channel of the Tiber), which was probably reduced to a one-man office by the Flavian period; oversight of the drains that fed the river was extended to the office by 100 CE, making the officer in charge the *curator alvei et riparum Tiberis et cloacarum urbis*.[31] The exact tasks of the *curator* are not entirely clear, but he probably marked the boundaries of the river, maintained the quays and cargo embankments (crucial for the importation of foodstuffs to the city), and organized efforts to prevent floods.[32] Romans thought it best to monitor and regulate rivers, not only in the vicinity of Rome but across the empire, given that rivers are not only great sources of public water, but also destructive agents.[33]

The administration and legal regulation of water in the city of Rome has been a subject of great interest since the beginning of the empire itself (particularly issues concerning the supply of water to the city). One of the best sources for reconstructing the *cura aquarum*, or the office in charge of water distribution, is Frontinus—a *curator* himself of the office. Reflecting on the past history of the office, Frontinus in *De aquaeductu urbis Romae* states that he wanted to provide a manual for his successor, and in the work, he covers

28 The Nile River's floods, for example, were famous for their life-giving and destructive properties. For more see Bonneau (1964, 29–131; 1993) and Campbell (2012, 136–37).

29 For an extensive discussion of the physical, social, and historical implications of Tiber River floods, see Aldrete (2007).

30 Aldrete 2007, 4–5.

31 Aldrete 2007, 199.

32 For an overview of the office, see Aldrete (2007, 198–203), Masi Doria and Cascione (2010), and Campbell (2012, 98–117). One can also refer to the *Lex de imperio Vespasiani* and its connection to river management; see Bruun (2012a). Campbell explores rivers in general throughout the Roman world, from practical matters, to wider cultural phenomena associated with these water sources (e.g., rivers in literature, religion, and art). See also the contributions in Franconi's 2017 volume on fluvial landscapes of the Roman world, including discussions of the impact of climate on rivers.

33 See the edited volume of Hermon (2010) that explores empire-wide issues of river control and other riparine issues.

numerous topics, such as the history of the aqueducts of Rome (including the actual capacities of each of the aqueducts), the distribution of private water rights from the emperor (addressing such details as the sizes of pipes, the *quinariae*), and various pieces of legislation (such as earlier *senatus consulta*) regarding water, amongst other smaller matters.

In addition to the inner workings of various aqueducts up to the early second century CE, Frontinus documents the imperial overhaul of the *cura aquarum*. The water administration office was probably set up after the aedileship of Agrippa in 33 BCE, who helped monumentalize Rome's water infrastructure on a scale far grander than anything seen in the Republic.[34] After Agrippa's death in 12 BCE, the administration was transferred to Augustus, who made it an office for those of senatorial rank through a *senatus consultum* of 11 BCE, as recorded and reported by Frontinus.[35] By the time of Frontinus, however, the office had apparently fallen into corruption and bad business practices. Frontinus, under the prerogative of the emperor, then continued to improve Rome's water supply, cracking down on illegal water tapping by private individuals. Using Frontinus' treatise, we know that the *curator*'s duties included:

> 1) The upkeep of the physical constructions necessary for the city's water supply, and, in doing so, to manage the work force at the disposition of the administration. 2) The registration of the private water grants. 3) Jurisdiction in a number of questions which concerned the aqueducts, such as infractions of private parties on the land reserved for the aqueducts.[36]

After Frontinus' time, the office of water administration continued to grow and transform, as exemplified by the creation of the office of the *curator aquarum et Minuciae*, or the office of water administration and grain distribution, two agencies that were merged in the early Severan period.[37] Frontinus also mentions that the organization of the *cura aquarum* included an architect (*architectus*), scribes (*scribae* and *librarii*), attendants (*accensi*), and heralds (*praecones*).[38] Oftentimes in modern literature, there is still some confusion

---

34 Bruun 1991, 140–52, especially 149; Peachin 2004, 82–138, especially 102–109.

35 Frontin. *Aq.* 100–101. See Peachin (2004, 103–104).

36 Bruun 1991, 183–84.

37 On this new office, see Taylor (2010).

38 Frontin. *Aq.* 100.1. There has been discussion on the exact location of the physical offices of the *cura aquarum* in the city of Rome. For the most recent evaluation, see Bruun (2007).

regarding the *aquarii*, which Frontinus uses a collective noun to denote the staff of the office (who were sometimes associated with selling water rights illegally), since the term can also refer to a class of professional water sellers, who would deliver water to Roman homes.[39] Further insight into the workings of the *cura aquarum* can be gained by comparing Frontinus' account with literary descriptions of other Roman administrative offices. For example, Jean-Jacques Aubert has compared the *cura aquarum* to the *vilicus* system (i.e., the management of an agricultural estate). Here, the estate owner (*dominus*) employed a *vilicus* (typically a slave or freedman) to organize farmwork and oversee his agricultural slaves. Likewise, the *curator aquarum* might hire someone (such as a *libertus* with procuratorial power) to manage the workforce of imperial slaves who performed regular maintenance on the water distribution network. Just as the *dominus'* slaves were legally considered part of his *familia*, so too could these imperial slaves be considered part of the *familia Caesaris*, as these properties were connected to the imperial family.[40]

Modern scholarship offers varying interpretive lenses for understanding Frontinus' *De aquaeductu*: as a literary work (Saastamoinen 2003, with both technical and rhetorical flourishes); as an incomplete treatise (Bruun 2003); as a speech perhaps read to the Senate (DeLaine 1996); as a panegyric for the emperor or Frontinus himself (Evans 1997).[41] Building on previous scholarship, Michael Peachin (2004) suggests that Frontinus was actually producing this work (and all of its details) to assert his power as *curator* and thereby persuade the incumbent aristocracy that the emperor's overhaul of Rome's water infrastructure would bring valuable benefits to the city. Whatever Frontinus' intentions may have been, his work is an important piece of evidence for understanding Roman water systems, especially aqueducts and related legislation until the early second century CE.

For reasons outlined above, Frontinus' *De aquaeductu* does not provide a complete or unbiased portrayal of Roman water systems; thankfully, however, archaeological evidence offers a different, complementary picture of Roman water administration. For example, some scholars have examined the engineering details mentioned in Frontinus (e.g., *calices*, the delivery necks of pipes, and the *quinaria*), which can provide insight into the amounts of water

39 Bruun 1991, 108–109, 190–94. See also Kehoe (2008), who discusses the impact related to the illegal selling of water on the Roman economy.

40 Aubert 1994, 323–24. See also De Kleijn (2001, 120–35).

41 See also, Blackman and Hodge's reappraisal of Frontinus (2001, 137–50).

flowing through the city and give some indications of population size.[42] More importantly, the stamps on lead pipes (*fistulae*) have helped modern scholars reconstruct the building programs and usage policies managed by the *cura aquarum*.[43] Christer Bruun (1991) used the *fistulae* found in Rome to illustrate who was installing water and who might have been using the water, given the names stamped on the pipes. Bruun demonstrates that, of the water coming into the city of Rome, 17% went to the emperor, 38% to private individuals, and 45% to the public at large.[44]

Bruun has also challenged prior understandings of *fistulae* in relation to water rights. In the past, *fistula* stamps have been used to reconstruct ownership of Rome's vast water network. Inscriptions on *fistulae* can be wide ranging: names of emperors; names of officials; names of individuals in the genitive case; names of individuals in the nominative case; consular dates; institution names; place of the conduit's manufacture; numbers; images; *miscellanea*.[45] It had been thought previously that a name in the genitive case appearing on a *fistula* stamp signified ownership of the water flowing through the pipes.[46] Bruun has rightly shown, however, that the genitive does not always indicate ownership, especially in the case of imperial names.[47] For example, a pipe labeled with an imperial name could mean that the water was supplying an imperial property (e.g., a bath complex) or a business related to the imperial *fiscus*, not simply supplying the emperor directly. Further, names on *fistulae* can indicate benefactions of the emperor, not necessarily ownership. *Fistulae* could also indicate the name of the pipe's manufacturer (or *plumbarius*, a person who specialized in metal product production).[48] Moreover, Gerda De Kleijn has argued that the available evidence for *fistula* stamps does not conclusively identify their meaning or role within the water infrastructure system,

42 Blackman and Hodge 2001; De Kleijn 2001, which provides conjectures about Rome's population, especially 68–74.

43 For more on the construction of lead pipes, see: Bruun 1991, 304–10; Cochet 2000, with previous bibliography; Jansen 2000c, 119–21; Hodge 2002, 307–15.

44 Bruun 1991, 63. Compare with the figures suggested by De Kleijn (2001, 69–70).

45 Bruun 2016b, 13–7. Prosopographic studies are also enriched by lead pipes, helping to fill in gaps of Italian families that might otherwise be unknown. For more, see Bruun (2012b).

46 Eck (1998) is a proponent of this interpretation.

47 Bruun 2001; Bruun 2016b, 17. See also De Kleijn's discussion of the problems of Bruun's previous scholarship before 2001, especially his 1991 monograph (2001, 115–20). Bruun's most recent article (2016b) succinctly lays out the current state of the field of *fistulae*.

48 For example, there is the case of a Stallianus found on lead pipe in the Stabian Baths at Pompeii, who might have been a *plumbarius*. See Bruun (2012d). Geremia Nucci (2006) documents the *plumbarii* of Ostia.

aside from conveying a general sense of control over the pipes and the water flowing through them.[49]

Much of the work to-date on Roman water administration (especially using archaeological evidence in conjunction with other literary sources) concerns the city of Rome itself, due in part to the prevalence of these pipes within the imperial capital. In fact, early in the study of *fistulae*, it was thought that only Rome had these types of inscriptions, but archaeological discoveries in the last few decades have shown that they were present throughout the empire, even though they might not appear with the same frequency.[50] For instance, while *fistula* stamps have been found concentrated in the city of Rome, they are also found in Ostia, Portus, the Bay of Naples, and some other sites on the Italian Peninsula.[51] Morever, because of the excellent state of Pompeii's preserved water infrastructure, this site has the potential to reveal logistics of Roman urban water management at a new level of detail.[52]

There has been a growing trend to examine, where possible, evidence of *fistulae* and other vestiges of the water distribution network outside of Rome, in order to obtain a fuller picture of Roman water administration at large. A 2006 conference at the Université Laval, "Vers une gestion intégrée de l'eau dans l'empire romain," drew a number of international scholars who presented archaeological, economic, and juridical evidence of water administration and usage across the empire.[53] This conference illustrates the need for cross-empire collaboration among scholars in order to create a diachronic, far-reaching geographic study of Roman water management systems.

Roman law is another important form of evidence for the administration, distribution, and regulation of water, both at Rome and throughout the

---

49 De Kleijn 2001, 138.

50 Bruun 2016b, 11–2.

51 The standard publication for the *fistulae* of Rome is still Heinrich Dressel's entries in the *CIL* (15.2.1, nos. 7235–7913). On Dressel and other early scholars of *fistulae*, see Bruun (2015a; 2016b, 11–3). For more on the find spots of the examples from the city of Rome, see Bruun (1991, 20–24; 2001, 55–8), Eck (1998), and De Kleijn (2001, 147–223). On Ostia, see Geremia Nucci (2001). Bruun in various publications covers the examples outside of Rome (1991, 272–303; 2001, 52–5; 2016b), including those of Campania (2010) and Pompeii (2012d); see also his cautionary note about what information can be used from the examples of Rome (2016b, 10). It should be noted that there was a diversity of materials used for water conduits throughout the empire: lead pipes in Rome and the Italian Peninsula; *tubuli*, which could be made in terracotta; other pipes could be constructed from wood or stone. For more, see De Kleijn (2001, 136), along with Jansen (2000c, especially 111–24).

52 On Pompeii's water private infrastructure, see Jansen (2001).

53 Hermon 2008.

empire. In the last two decades, scholars of Roman law have begun to shed light on the legal regulation of water, providing a more nuanced understanding of water usage and access to water sources, especially in terms of private water rights. Of course, government regulation of water systems (or concerted efforts to control water by those in power) has been present since prehistory, as evidenced in Mesopotamia, the Arabian Peninsula, and Egypt.[54] Whereas local laws throughout the Greek world generally construed a basic right to water for all people (e.g., the right to use a neighbor's water if one does not have any), Roman law is explicit in differentiating between public and private water rights.[55] The latter was determined in strict connection to the land on which the water rests (rather than on an individual or family basis). And while publicly-owned water assured that all people had access to water, the principles underlying these legal distinctions overcame the 'tragedy of the commons' (by which individuals tend to consume as much as possible of a common resource because no individual gains by saving or investing for the future).[56] In a sense, at least part of the Roman water supply was privately owned, which guaranteed individual interest in maintaining sound water management policies.

Although a full examination of Roman policies associated with water cannot be offered here, some salient points will be made, in order to show how Roman law constructed principles of water access for inhabitants across the empire. Scholars draw on a wide range of evidence to demonstrate Roman legal thinking about water, from inscriptions (e.g., laws and legal contracts), juridical texts, and literary sources.[57] Romans were especially concerned that water systems be protected in order to safeguard healthy water supplies, both in and outside urban centers.[58] To this end, much of Roman law focuses on controlling access to water throughout its journey across rural aqueducts (which individuals might tap for private use) to its final distribution within an

54 Bruun 2000.

55 For more on the differences between Greek and Roman conceptions of water access, see Bruun (2000, 557–604). On Greek water legal practices, especially through the works of Plato and Aristotle, see Louis (1982). See above, 10–11, on public and private waters in Roman law.

56 On the modern theory of the 'tragedy of the commons,' see Ostrom (1990).

57 Again, the bibliography on this subject is vast. Some key works to consult are Shaw (1982), Bruun (2000, 575–604; 2015b), Bannon (2001; 2009; 2013), and Kehoe (2008). Difficulties arise in Roman legal documents concerning with water, as it is believed that many water-related cases were done by case law, until full codification of Roman law occurred in the sixth century CE (Wilson 2012, 4; below, 60).

58 Bruun 2000, 592–95; Taylor 2000, 87–92; Taylor 2009, 31–6.

urban destination.[59] Thus, like much of Roman life, there is a clear dichotomy between rural and urban water rights, predicated on the intended use of the water (e.g., for use in crop irrigation versus bath complexes).

In rural Roman areas, there were two methods to gain access to water: through cooperative community agreements and servitudes. There is evidence, for example, in the semi-arid and arid climates of North Africa, that communities would come together to form agreements on how to share water sources, usually for the irrigation of agricultural lands. At Lamasba in Numidia (modern Algeria) around 212–218 CE, multiple communities collectively formulated a plan to distribute water on a schedule to different farmsteads. This program was overseen by a board of three that represented the settlements' decurions and citizens.[60] Although this example, along with many others, was inscribed, no doubt similar arrangements were also devised as simple oral agreements between various parties.[61] Regardless, such cooperation among rural communities appears to have been commonplace throughout the Roman Empire, illustrating a relatively consistent pattern in social resolutions to the practical problems of rural water supply.[62]

On the Italian Peninsula, in order to obtain access to another's private water supply, an individual had to obtain a servitude.[63] As part of the *iura praediorum*, rustic or predial (or property-related) servitudes were often permanent mechanisms through which one could access a neighbor's property and its resources, such as water.[64] Rustic servitudes related to water included the *servitus aquae ductus* (the ability to channel water) and the *servitus aquae haustus* (the ability to draw water).[65] Thus, if one did not have a natural water source on their own land, he or she could make a contract with a neighbor, in order to obtain access to their water for private use, including agricultural irrigation.

59 For more on the use of water from aqueducts going through the countryside, see Wilson (1999).

60 *CIL* 8.18587 = 4440 = *ILS* 5793. Shaw 1982; Meuret 1996; Kehoe 2008, 246–47; Bannon 2009, 76–7; Bruun 2015b, 142–43.

61 Shaw 1982, 68.

62 Bruun 2015b; 144. Another commonly cited example is the cooperative arrangement of the inhabitants alongside the Ebro River in Spain during the reign of Hadrian, the *lex rivi Hiberiensis*. For more, see the initial publication by Beltrán Lloris (2006), along with subsequent discussions by Kehoe (2008, 244) and Bruun (2015b, 145).

63 Servitudes seem to only be operational on the Italian Peninsula. See Bruun (2015b, 147).

64 In English, servitudes are often known as 'easements' in modern legal terminology. On servitudes generally, with a helpful bibliography, see Bannon (2009, especially 12, note 33), along with Bruun (2000, 581–85; 2015b, 145–49).

65 Bannon 2009, 13. See also Kehoe (2008, 245).

Water servitudes in rural areas, as Cynthia Bannon argues, promoted a competitiveness and cooperation within communities that aided in their economic success.[66] Bruun, however, disagrees with some of Bannon's conclusions; he argues that Bannon has conflated servitudes with other water-sharing arrangements, since only servitudes addressed individual properties and issues of private ownership.[67] Indeed, instances of cooperation between communities dealing with public water sources were often temporary, not permanent like servitudes.[68]

While servitudes were used in cities, civic legal policies regulated private water access in the urban sphere more often than individual servitudes. For example, outside Rome, there is clear epigraphic evidence for private water rights that must have been granted by local town councils (rather than the emperor).[69] In the city of Rome, private water access could be granted through the *beneficium* of the emperor, often via the *cura aquarum*. Dennis Kehoe has argued that at Rome, where demand for access to water was astronomically high, grants of private water rights often became corrupt, tapping more water than legally permitted at the expense of public supplies, creating an underground market in which water distribution did not economically benefit *all* of the inhabitants of Rome.[70]

Considering the great need for public water, an important issue for the Roman state was the acquisition of land for the construction of public aqueducts. Rabun Taylor's 2000 study of the aqueducts of Rome outlines the evidence as to how the Romans constructed aqueducts. Taylor is emphatic that the Roman state did not expropriate land for aqueducts, but instead purchased land (or in the very least servitudes), presumably at market value.[71] Among the evidence that Taylor cites, the course of the Aqua Virgo, built by Agrippa, does not follow a simple westerly path, but snakes north and south, perhaps responding to landowners not honoring agreements with Agrippa to allow the construction of the aqueduct on their land.[72] Indeed, Taylor points out that

---

66 Bannon 2009.

67 Bruun 2015b, 146.

68 Bruun 2015b, 147. There could be lapses in the rights to a servitude, however, as some had to be exercised within two years of an agreement or only for a certain period of time. For more, see Bannon (2009, 18–9) and Bruun (2015b, 149). See also Bannon (2013) for a discussion of legal issues related to water piping on properties being sold to another party.

69 Bruun 2015b, 135.

70 Kehoe 2008, 244–45.

71 Taylor 2000, 93–127. Taylor reacts to de Robertis' 1936 study that argued that Roman law allowed for land expropriation.

72 Taylor 2000, 104.

Roman law emphasized ownership above all else, making expropriation of lands impossible.[73] Not all scholars, however, agree with this position. Bruun argues that the Romans expropriated not only the land on which aqueducts were constructed, but also the land surrounding these monumental waterways, in order to use its material resources for necessary aqueduct repairs.[74]

While the primary and secondary literature on Roman water administration, distribution, and legal practices is vast and complex, this brief discussion has illustrated a few salient points about its organization and basic principles: (1) The administration of water in the city of Rome itself and throughout the empire was meant to provide all inhabitants, especially those in arid and semi-arid climates, access to potable water. (2) There are clear distinctions in types of water access, whether public or private, rural or urban. Roman legal policies concerning water are crucial to understanding the relationship between the Roman economy and law, especially for rural Roman life. (3) Further, scholars continue to expand investigations beyond the evidence from the city of Rome itself, stretching to the boundaries of the empire, in order to clarify the powerful mechanisms through which the Roman Empire achieved the goal of providing water to all of its inhabitants.

4 Categories of Water Usage: Archaeological Evidence

Archaeological evidence of Roman water structures is the foundation of any full, nuanced understanding of Roman water culture. Classical archaeologists have been fascinated with Roman water structures for the last century or so; therefore, these structures are often featured in the wider discourse of Roman culture. In the last few decades, however, numerous archaeological discoveries and investigations have not only expanded modern conceptions of Roman water usage, but have also challenged previously held opinions and altered preconceived notions. Among the archaeological evidence explored in this section are aqueducts, baths, drainage and sanitation, water-displays, and hydraulic power.

---

73 Taylor, on the one hand, demonstrates that 'expropriation' is not a Roman legal concept in and of itself, and the notion of 'eminent domain' is a Medieval legal coinage. Confiscation, on the other hand, is based on consequences of an individual's actions, such as a criminal act. See Taylor (2000, 93–4).

74 Bruun 2000, 595–98. Bruun uses the example of the 11 BCE *senatus consultum* cited in Frontinus (124.4–125), which gives those workers the ability to seize materials.

A brief note must be mentioned, however, concerning an important theme that will resurface over and over throughout the ensuing discussion. One of the major issues when exploring the use of water in the Roman Empire is the dichotomy between public and private use. Andrea Schmölder-Veit, working primarily on fountains in the western empire, suggests using categories of water usage, based on Latin terminologies:[75] *utilitas* (utility), *usus* (consumption), *salubritas* (cleanliness), *salus* (health), *voluptas/amoenitas* (beauty). She asserts that conceptions of water in the public sphere are related to *utilitas, usus, salubritas*, and *salus*, while private life is related to *voluptas/amoenitas*. But one could easily argue that all of these terms are crucial to both public and private use and needs. While there are differences between public and private water-related structures (e.g., scale), there are nevertheless overlapping interests between the two spheres, which must be remembered.

4.1 *Prolegomena: Modern Scholarship on Roman Water*

Before outlining the major categories of water usage, it is important to highlight some organizations that promote the study of Roman water systems. Many of the scholars responsible for publishing water-related archaeological evidence are also active members of the Deutsche Wasserhistorische Gesellschaft, the Frontinus Gesellschaft, and other international organizations. It is crucial first to survey their scholarly activities, which will lay a strong foundation for the ensuing discussion.

The Deutsche Wasserhistorische Gesellschaft (DWhG) is a German society that promotes the study of water in all time periods.[76] The current society was founded in 2002. Originally, however, the society was formed by Martin Eckoldt in 1963 as the Bundesanstalt für Gewässerkunde, which would go on to organize the "Geschichte und Zukunft einer wasserhistorischen Kongress-Serie," a series of international symposia held every few years. Until 1991, the symposia were organized by Günther Garbrecht and Henning Fahlbusch in coorperation of the *Leichtweiß-Institut für Wasserbau* of the Technischen Universität Braunschweig.[77] After the 1991 symposium, the series took on the title *Cura*

75 Schmölder-Veit 2009, 23–5.

76 http://www.dwhg-ev.de/index.html (Last accessed 10 September 2017).

77 The symposia were held in: Koblenz 1975; Lyon 1977; Istanbul 1979; Athens 1981; Jerusalem 1983; Cairo 1985; Rome 1988; Mérida 1991. Many of them were subsequently published by the Institute: Istanbul 1979; Athens 1981; Jerusalem 1984; Cairo 1986; Rome 1989; Mérida 1992.

Aquarum, which is still active today.[78] Many of the publications of the *Cura Aquarum* series illustrate the breadth and sweep of Roman water technology and its implementation throughout the Roman world. Readers can simply browse through the titles to find interesting articles, with new archaeological data and methodological approaches.

The Frontinus Gesellschaft, founded in 1976, is another German organization that is concerned with the history of water technology and usage, particularly in the Roman period.[79] Named after Sextus Julius Frontinus, the organization brings together scholars from a variety of disciplines (e.g., Classics, Engineering, Archaeology) at a variety of conferences and excursions, the latter promoting on-site autopsy. In addition, the society has an annual journal (*Schriftenreihe der Frontinus Gesellschaft*), a series on water supply (*Geschichte der Wasserversorgung*), and a supplemental series, which often stems from the society's conferences.[80] While this organization is largely comprised of German-speaking scholars, their meetings include a growing number of international researchers.

Recently, a handful of international research networks have formed to study water in the ancient Mediterranean. The HYDRΩMED Project, based at the University of Aix-Marseille (France), has explored water management in the Mediterranean during the first millennium BCE through a series

78 The symposia associated with the *Cura Aquarum* series include: Pompeii (Campania) 1994; Syracuse, Sicily 1998; Jerusalem, Israel 2001; Ephesus 2004; Jordan 2007; Toledo, Spain 2009; Jerusalem 2012; Athens 2015. To-date the following symposia have been published: Pompeii 1996; Sicily 2000; Israel 2002; Ephesus 2006; Jordan 2008; Athens 2017. See Koloski-Ostrow et al., (1997) for a review of the 1996 proceedings, along with Koloski-Ostrow (2008) on the 2006 proceedings. It must be noted that the *Cura Aquarum* series was a joint collaboration between the DWhG and the Frontinus Gesellschaft; however, after 2006, due to a legal dispute, the DWhG took over the series.

79 http://www.frontinus.de/index.html (Last accessed 10 September 2017). While much of the activity of the society is focused on the Roman period, the group still promotes water history in subsequent periods—all the way to the Baroque period. For example, in their publication series, *Geschichte der Wasserversorgung*, they have published on the Middle Ages (Band 4, 1991; Band 7, 2007), the Renaissance (Band 5, 2000), and the Baroque period (Band 6, 2004).

80 The ancient period titles of the *Geschichte der Wasserversorgung* series include: ancient Rome (Band 1, 1986; with a second edition, 2013) and the ancient cities (Band 2, 1987, including Pergamon, legislation, fountains, and building elements; Band 3, 1988, including baths and hygiene). Conference proceedings include one on ancient baths (Kreiner and Letzner 2012), historical water systems (Wiplinger 2013), Frontinus' legacy in Asia Minor (Wiplinger 2016b), and water management in the time of Frontinus (Wiplinger and Letzner 2017).

of conferences.[81] At a meeting in Athens in July 2015, the project presented "Water Cult and Culture in the Mediterranean World of the 1st Millennium BC," providing a number of papers that explored the implications of water in cultic settings of Greece and beyond. The Idraulica Antica: Gruppo di Studio Sull'Idraulica Antica, based at the University of Padova (Italy), brings together international scholars to discuss matters not only concerning Roman hydraulic systems, but also the implications of water on Roman urban and social landscapes.[82] The group has hosted a series of international summer schools in the nearby town of Feltre, on the following topics: Hydraulic Systems in the Roman World (2014); Water and the City: Hydraulic Systems in the Roman Age (2015); Water Management in Arid and Semiarid Climates in Roman Times (2016). In November 2017, a conference also took place at Feltre, "Water and the Roman Cities and Settlements."

The *Aquae Urbis Romae*, or the "The Waters of the City of Rome," project of Katherine Rinne is an important online resource for all scholars on the use of water in the city from its founding until the present day.[83] This site houses information on the complex water infrastructure of Rome, which allows scholars to see exactly how the use of water has evolved. The project also includes a journal, *The Waters of Rome*, which publishes online refereed papers that explore issues related to water in Rome from antiquity to the present.

The journal *Water History* explores all time periods of humans' use of water—attempting to understand how water has influenced human communities.[84] With the proliferation of modern water-related problems across the globe, studying water systems of the past has become all the more relevant. Today, the world is faced with issues of water access, the commodification of water, and the destructive properties of water. A number of organizations study water management, safeguards for water, and hydro-environmental sciences in general, such as the programs of UNESCO.[85] And just as the past can inform

81 Sophie Bouffier, a professor at University of Aix-Marseille, coordinates the project. The network's website is: http://hydromed.hypotheses.org/ (Last accessed 10 September 2017).

82 The group's coordinator is Prof. Paola Zanovello at the University of Padova. For more, see the group's website: https://idraulicantica.wordpress.com/ (Last accessed 10 September 2017).

83 Rinne 2016.

84 Of special interest here, however, are two special issues: "Roman and Byzantine Empires" (Vol. 4.1, 2012) and "Roman Canals" (Vol. 6.1, 2014).

85 Bibliography on modern issues associated with water is immense. One can easily consult the studies of Strang (2004; 2006; 2008; 2012), whose research investigates not only humans' experience with water, but also the cultural significance of water in modern life. The water-related programs of UNESCO, such as the International Hydrological Program,

our interpretation of present water crises, so too can these modern cases help us think about how the Romans used and manipulated water.

4.2 *Aqueducts and Water Supply Systems*

One of the most enduring examples of Roman engineering ingenuity was its ability to move and store water on a massive scale. Before the Roman aqueduct, there were many ways in which water collection was facilitated (and even continued after the advent of the canonical Roman aqueduct building form): wells, cisterns, tunnels, *qanats*, etc.[86] While the Romans certainly did not invent the aqueduct by any means, they were able to incorporate new technologies and scales of building, such as:

> the use of arcades to carry channels over valleys and low-lying terrain; the availability of concrete as a cheap and adaptable building material; the adoption of waterproof cement linings from the Punic world or Hellenistic Sicily; the expanded use of lead piping and of bronze stopcocks on distribution systems; and the introduction of settling tanks and storage and reservoirs on the network.[87]

Aqueducts in particular were great feats of engineering that funneled water from natural sources (e.g., springs or rivers) into large conduits, which simply relied on gravity to move water.

---

seek to promote the management of natural water resources throughout the world (to secure necessary freshwater) and safeguard water security to ensure that all have access to water. (See: http://www.unesco.org/new/en/natural-sciences/environment/water/; (Last accessed 10 September 2017)) The question of who owns water is especially divisive as water can be considered a commodity, which can limit the ability to retrieve water. Further, there are conferences, such as in 2011 at the University of Pennsylvania, that explore the modern terrain of water. The Pennsylvania meeting explored the notion of how water can be conceptualized intellectually, or it can have a physical presence, drastically altering landscapes and human lives (Mathur and da Cuhna 2014). See also Black (2016) for a succinct overview of issues related to modern water resources.

86 For more on precursors to Roman aqueducts, see: Tölle-Kastenbein 1990, 21–42; Crouch 1993; Tölle-Kastenbein 1994; Hodge 2002, 19–47; Wilson 2008, 290–96. On wells and cisterns, see overviews by Brinker (1990), Riera (1994, 297–388), Hodge (2000c, 29–34; 2002, 48–66), and Wilson (2008, 285–90); on tunnels, see especially Grewe (1998; 2008). The *qanat* is an underground water-tunnel system that is popular in the Middle East and some parts of North Africa. For a brief overview, see Hodge (2000b, 35–38), along with Wilson (2009).

87 Wilson 2008, 296.

A majority of Roman aqueducts were simple channels often constructed with masonry blocks.[88] These channels followed the natural contours of the land, and they were installed 50 cm to 1 m below the surface of the earth, making them easy to install and maintain over time. The masonry channels themselves were generally tall and oblong (to allow for easy cleaning and maintence by work crews), lined with waterproof cement, and were probably half to two-thirds full of water when operational.[89] Other forms of channels included open channels (taking advantage of rock formations) and piping systems (using terracotta, lead, stone, and wood).[90] When Roman engineers could not use subterranean aqueduct systems, they relied on various engineering works, including grander tunnel systems, emabankments, bridges/viaducts, siphons, and continuous arcades.[91] Inverted siphons, which are often found in Gaul, allowed water to cross valleys, in which an aqueduct entered a header tank at one side of the valley, and then continued down the slope in pipes, where the resulting pressure would push the water to the receiving tank on the opposite side of the valley.[92] Arcades provided raised surfaces for aqueduct channels to travel (especially across plains), allowing for the necessary changes in gradient to provide sufficient water pressure at the terminus.[93] Although arcades associated with aqueducts are not nearly as numerous as subterranean channels, the aesthetic rhythm of their arches stretching across the landscape has become an iconic representation of Romans' ability to harness natural forces.[94]

Not all aqueducts lead to Rome, however. Aqueduct systems had various destinations. Aqueducts supplied mining operations throughout the Roman world,[95] as well as hundreds of military camps.[96] Moreover, Harry Evans has demonstrated how the aqueducts running through the Tiburtine region toward Rome also included extensions that served various rural communities.[97] These communities included villas and farms, which needed a great deal of water to sustain the agricultural and industrial activities. In addition to

88 Hodge 2002, 93.

89 Hodge 2002, 94–5.

90 Hodge 2002, 105–17.

91 Hodge 2002, 126–70.

92 Hodge 2002, 147–60. See Wilson (2002, 295–96) on the Hellenistic precursors of the Roman siphon.

93 Hodge 2002, 161–70.

94 For more on the symbolic character of the architecture of Roman aqueducts, see Kek (1996, especially 265–316).

95 See Wilson 2002.

96 See, for example, Fevrier (1983).

97 Evans 1993.

aqueducts, these people relied on other water systems, such as ground water, rainwater runoff, and irrigation systems.[98]

Aqueducts also supplied urban centers, but they did not act alone. They were part of a larger urban supply network.[99] When water entered a city, it would generally pass first through the *castellum aquae/divisorium*, which, in turn, would supply the water to specific areas of urban space. Two well preserved examples are found at Nîmes and Pompeii, both of which are tripartite, allowed the water to be distributed in three different ways; exactly which parts of the city were supplied by these divisions has been a matter of debate since antiquity.[100] Water then travelled throughout the Roman town and supplied a number of consumers: public baths, public fountains, industrial complexes, private dwellings, etc. Private water connections are well understood, thanks in part to the evidence from Pompeii, with nearly 124 private connections found.[101] Water inside the home, according to the evidence from Pompeii, could be controlled easily, as it entered the home through lead pipes, travelled through a distribution box, which could be shut off using taps and stopcocks.[102] The use of lead pipes in water distribution has led some scholars to attribute the decline of the Roman Empire to lead poisoning, a conclusion that has been repeatedly refuted in the last few decades.[103]

---

98 For more on these systems, especially in Latium and south Etruria, see Thomas and Wilson (1994). See Wilson (2008, 309–10) on irrigation systems. For more on the role of aqueducts in the countryside, see Wilson (1999), along with his work on the impact of both climate change and drought on North African agricultural irrigation systems (2017).

99 For more on urban distribution of water, see: Jansen 2000c, 111–25; Hodge 2002, 273–303; Wilson 2008, 302–304.

100 Vitruvius, on the one hand, states that the *castellum* would provide water for the baths, public fountains, and private water connections in the city (*De arch.* 8.6.2). Frontinus, on the other hand, states that the water would be for public, private, and imperial use (*Aq.* 3.2). Ohlig has shown through the *castellum* example at Pompeii that Vitruvius is incorrect in his assertion, as the conduits from the *castellum* do not supply just baths, fountains, and domestic spaces (Ohlig 1995, 135–40; Ohlig 2001). Hodge reminds the reader that Vitruvius is not an encyclopedia or a strict how-to-guide, but a recommendation for the reader (2002, 282). For more on the *castellum aquae*, see Hodge (2002, 291–303).

101 Jansen (2001) presents one of the first systematic studies of domestic water supply. See now Dessales (2013, 179–224), who offers an even fuller discussion of the elements of domestic water systems there.

102 For more on Roman water taps, see Kretzschmer (1960), Balty (1962), Lebel (1965), and Jansen (2001, 29–31).

103 Among the proponents of lead poisoning in the Roman Empire are Gilfillan (1965) and Nriagu (1983). In addition to lead being found in piping for water, lead was also present in a number of other products that Romans consumed, including some cosmetics

The topic of Roman water supply has been studied in earnest for the past century to varying degrees of detail, with different emphases. The city of Rome itself had 11 different aqueducts, with its first in 312 BCE, the Aqua Appia, and the last in 226 CE, the Aqua Alexandrina.[104] The first modern treatises on these 11 aqueducts were by Esther Van Deman (1934) and Thomas Ashby (1935), who both examined the standing remains of the structures, providing important observations and photographic evidence from the early twentieth century of structures that have not all survived to present day. Until Van Deman and Ashby, the aqueducts of Rome had not been systematically studied, a point that Ashby bemoans in his preface.[105]

Since the pioneering work of Ashby and Van Deman, scholars have worked tirelessly to study specific aqueduct systems. Klaus Grewe in 1986 published the aqueduct of Köln in a monograph that explored not only the aqueduct itself, but also the engineering issues of the structure. The aqueduct of Nîmes and the associated Pont du Gard were first published extensively in 1991 by a French team, who then published a second edition in 2000.[106] The importance of this work lies in the breadth of expertise that the contributing scholars collectively used to examine the aqueduct, in terms of its actual structure, its placement in the landscape, and its impact on the urban settlement of Nîmes. Other studies of note include the aqueducts of Spain (especially Segovia),[107]

---

and sweeteners. Vitruvius (*De arch.* 8.6.10–11) and Pliny the Elder (*HN* 34.50.167) knew of the potential dangers to humans of lead usage. For a pointed critique of Nriagu, see Scarborough (1984). Current archaeological and osteological research demonstrates that there certainly was lead consumption by the Romans (and could be dangerous in and of itself), but not on the level that would cause the decline of a whole empire. For more, see Keenan-Jones, Hellstrom, and Drysdale (2011) and Delile et al. (2014). For an overview of lead poisoning throughout history, see Lessler (1988). Waters contaminated with lead are still a problem today. The World Health Organization's International Program on Chemical Safety still monitors lead usage and actively promotes the discontinuation of lead in products that are consumed.

104 The 11 aqueducts are: Appia (312 BCE); Vetus (272–269 BCE); Marcia (144–140 BCE); Tepula (126–125 BCE); Julia (33 BCE); Virgo (22–19 BCE); Alesietina (2 BCE); Claudia and Anio Novus (finished in 52 CE); Traiana (109); Alexandrina (226). For more on the chronology and construction of the aqueducts of Rome, see: Aicher 1995, 31–45; Taylor 2000; Koloski-Ostrow 2001, 5–6; Bianco 2007, 19–67; Wilson 2008, 296–97.

105 Ashby 1935, ix.

106 Fabre, Fiches, and Paillet 2000.

107 An early overview of the Roman aqueducts of Spain can be found in Fernández Casado (1972); on the Segovia aqueduct, see Mas-Guindal Lafarga (1992).

Pergamon,[108] Ephesus,[109] and Athens.[110] Many of the scholars who publish on aqueducts are French and German, probably due to the fact that they were the first to examine these ancient structures in their native countries. But more recently, studies of aqueducts located in other countries, produced by a more international group of scholars, have been cropping up, notably in Israel and Greece.[111] Furthermore, new research is being conducted on previously excavated aqueduct systems (such as at Ostia), as well as recently discovered sources and their conduits (such as the head of the Aqua Traiana near Lake Bracciano, north of Rome).[112] One can easily find individual reports on aqueducts and their water systems throughout the Roman world in the various publications of the *Cura Aquarum* series.

While scholars have continued to document individual aqueduct systems, it is important to note that, by the 1980s, a shift in interpretive approach had occurred: a move away from traditional, detailed analyses of individual aqueducts toward more comparative, diachronic studies of aqueducts across the empire. In 1977, a conference in Lyon brought French and German scholars together to discuss not only aqueducts in France, but also Pompeii, Carthage, Attica, Pergamon, Trier, and Algeria, among a few others.[113] While individual sites are singled out within this volume, bringing them together in one place allowed for a new comparative approach across a wide swath of geography. Then, in the late 1980s, the Frontinus Gesellschaft produced two volumes (as

---

108 Garbrecht 2001.

109 Wiplinger 2016a. Wiplinger has spent much of his career investigating the aqueducts of Ephesus.

110 Leigh 1998. See also Leigh (2001) about early Roman hydraulic systems in Athens, along with her study of the reservoir of Hadrian in Athens (1997). For more on the development of Athenian water infrastructure systems from the Hellenistic period until the nineteenth century, see Christaki et al. (2017a), and from the nineteenth century until the present, see Christaki et al. (2017b).

111 On aqueducts in Israel, see Amit, Patrich, and Hirschfeld (2002). New research is coming out of Greece through the 2015 *Cura Aquarum* symposium in Athens (Wellbrock 2017), Giorgi's 2016 study of the Byzantine aqueduct of Gortyn (Crete), Vitti's 2016 study of vaulting construction in the Peloponnese that also discusses vaulted the aqueduct channels of Argos and Corinth, and an edited volume on *Great Waterworks in Roman Greece* (Aristodemou and Tassios 2018). See also Kamash (2010, 99–112) for more on water supply of the Roman Near East.

112 See Bukowiecki, Dessales, and Dublouloz (2008) for their work on the water systems of Ostia. Taylor et al. (2016) have been working over the last few years documenting the until now unknown parts of the Aqua Traiana located near its source.

113 Boucher 1983. Of interest, see Fevrier's chapter on the role of the Roman military and the construction of aqueducts.

part of its *Geschichte der Wasserversorgung* series) that examine aqueducts more holistically, whether by investigating water systems and distribution networks in general, or by studying the social implications of aqueducts.[114] In both volumes, close attention was paid to the structures associated with water distribution systems at a number of sites throughout the Roman world, from the northern provinces to the eastern provinces—in a way not seen until that point. In the second volume, Werner Eck provides one of the first systematic and prolonged discussions of the social implications of water distribution in the Roman city, suggesting the elevated status of a settlement that boasted its own water distribution network.[115]

In 1987, a colloquium was held in New York aptly titled, "Future Currents in Aqueduct Studies." The published proceedings contained important contributions for the study of Roman aqueducts. Philippe Leveau provides a synthesis of the preceding ten years of research on aqueducts, particularly in examining how architecture (i.e., water systems) impacts socio-economic systems.[116] Brent Shaw, using evidence from North Africa, also presents new ideas: interpreting water systems as status symbols and aqueducts as both objects of utility and luxury; demonstrating how members of the local élite maintained aqueduct systems; and further investigating the dichotomy of rural and urban water collection and distribution.[117] A. Trevor Hodge, the editor of the volume, asserts that there needs to be more emphasis on the engineering and technological aspects of Roman water supply, since, more often than not, classicists and archaeologists do not have the relevant engineering background to sufficiently evaluate this aspect of the water supply.[118]

After this colloquium was published, Hodge's seminal work was released in 1992, *Roman Aqueducts and Water Supply*. Immediately it became a standard text regarding aqueducts, made even more accessible for the first time in English, unlike previous scholarship which tended to primarily be in German. Picking up from his own suggestion in 1991, here Hodge includes lengthy discussions of the more technological aspects of the Roman water supply—giving

114 *Wassersorgung* II (1987) and *Wasserversorgung* III (1988). The second volume was released in a second edition in 2013.

115 Eck 1987.

116 Leveau 1991. He divided his discussion into the following sections: the archaeology of aqueducts (their architecture; how they function); social and economic conditions (cost; duration and organization of work); aqueducts and civilization (aqueducts as public monuments; their role in urban water supply).

117 Shaw 1991.

118 Hodge 1991.

his reader a more complete understanding of how a Roman aqueduct actually functioned. A second edition was released in 2002 without substantial changes, but with a supplemental bibliography, making the work still an invaluable resource.

During the 1990s, work continued on aqueducts in general. In *Utilitas necessaria: Sistemi idraulici nell'Italia romana* (1994), Giulio Bodon, Italo Riera, and Paola Zanovello thoroughly present the evidence for aqueducts and water systems in Italy, making their volume a cornerstone of research on regional trends within the empire.[119] Peter Aicher's 1995 guide to the aqueducts of Rome was an important update to the work of Ashby and Van Deman, helping the modern visitor to Rome understand the aqueducts (especially when the previous guides had been rendered obsolete with subsequent destruction of those structures). Another French conference in 1996, following in the footsteps of Boucher, presented new information on aqueducts in Gaul and further afield.[120] Roger Wilson, in a state of the field essay of 1996, points out the important work done on Roman water supply systems, including the monographs on specific aqueducts. Wilson, however, also stressed the work being done on private aqueducts that are present throughout the Roman world—illustrating archaeological evidence that is not always on the forefront of scholarship.

In the late 1990s, the debate on the actual purpose of aqueducts grew, especially through the work of Andrew Wilson. Although most scholars simply stressed the luxurious aspects of aqueducts (as they were objects of benefaction, either from the emperor or members of the local élite),[121] taking note of Brent Shaw's study of North Africa, Wilson instead stresses the utilitarian nature of aqueducts. In a sense, he wants others to consider the aqueducts in the wider water supply system—particularly systems that are outside of urban centers, which would have served large populations and supplied agricultural estates.[122] In the same vein as Wilson, Ann Koloski-Ostrow, in her 2001 edited volume, *Water Use and Hydraulics in the Roman City*, which started with a panel at the 1996 annual meeting of the Archaeological Institute of America, also stresses the need to investigate aqueducts as one part of a wider water supply and distribution network, in which all of the requisite parts work together to supply the ancient Roman town with sufficient water. This collected volume paid special attention to Pompeii, an important site for understanding water supply systems, particularly given the available archaeological evidence

119 See especially Riera (1994, 165–296) on aqueducts, along with Wilson (2000b, 597).

120 Bedon 1997.

121 See especially Wilson 1998.

122 Thomas and Wilson 1994; Wilson 1999.

of the *castellum aquae*, the water towers, along with street fountains and private water connections throughout the city.

The last decade also has seen an increase of scholars investigating water supply with an emphasis on technology and engineering principles. Örjan Wikander's *Handbook of Ancient Water Technology* (2000) is an important collection of essays from leading scholars that illustrate the various principles of water supply in the Mediterranean basin (from the Bronze Age to the Greco-Roman period). John Peter Oleson in 2008 presented an edited volume on various themes of engineering principles in the Greco-Roman world, which included water supply among other diverse topics, such as agriculture and warfare. Thus, water supply in the modern scholarship has been approached from various angles, including studies of aqueducts themselves, the wider water distribution networks, the social implications of aqueducts and water supply, and the technological aspects of these structures.

Conferences, of course, still continue to promote the study of individual aqueducts and larger water supply systems. In 2009, a French conference, *Les réseaux d'eau courante dans l'antiquité*, explored both aqueducts in France and some other locations, in addition to other hydraulic networks outside of France.[123] The Frontinus Gesellschaft's 2011 international symposium examined historical water systems, including sites in Germany, Turkey, Spain, and even South America (Brazil).[124] A particularly interesting discovery presented at these proceedings is the use of sinter (the calcium carbonate sediment that builds up in aqueduct channels) in determining the date of an aqueduct with a relatively high degree of accuracy.[125] Such research illustrates the continued need for interdisciplinary approaches to the study of aqueducts.

In the last decade, studies have continued the endeavor to place aqueducts and other water-related structures more meaningfully within the broader contexts of landscape and water supply networks. For example, Julian Richard makes the case for connecting specific fountains to the respective aqueducts that once supplied them.[126] Monuments, as Richard argues, should not be seen in isolation, but as a part of a larger network of water, particularly as flowing water gave these structures vitality and meaning. In the same vein, Elisabetta Giorgi traces the impact of the aqueduct of Gortyn (Crete) throughout the city's history, highlighting the numerous aspects of urban life that depended

123 Abadie-Reynal, Provost, and Vipard 2011.

124 Wiplinger 2011.

125 Sürmelihindi and Passchier 2011.

126 Richard 2012, 47–92.

on water resources supplied by this aqueduct.[127] Giorgi also investigates the relationship of Gortyn's aqueduct with its surrounding landscape, which is often missing in modern scholarship.

There are plenty of salient points to glean from past studies of Roman aqueducts—and also many future avenues of inquiry. The publication of individual aqueduct systems (whether initial or subsequent studies) is still vital. These, in turn, can be pulled together to form regional studies of aqueduct and water system usage throughout the Roman world. Next, the call for interdisciplinary studies of water systems is being fulfilled—with scholars incorporating engineering and scientific analyses to obtain the full picture of the nuanced intricacies of Roman aqueducts. Finally, there has been a rise of scholars placing aqueducts into wider water supply networks, focusing on their final destinations (whether urban or extra-urban), as well as their impact on such communities. In the future, it would be a *desideratum* to have an updated synthetic and diachronic analysis of aqueducts and water supply systems throughout the Roman Empire (perhaps as an updated version of Hodge's study), which not only pulls together new evidence from various parts of the Roman world, but also places aqueducts in a wider social network, stressing the socio-economic implications of Roman water usage practices.[128]

4.3 *Baths*

One of the most enduring aspects of Roman water culture is perhaps the phenomenon of the Roman bath. Romans are often credited with creating a more hygienic lifestyle; however, as modern scholarship has begun to demonstrate, bathing in a similar manner to the Romans was already popular in Greek culture and bathing was not as 'clean' as modern hygienic standards would demand. Regardless, bathing was omnipresent throughout the Roman world, using similar technologies to allow for heated water for relaxing bathing experiences. This section explores precursors to Roman baths, technical aspects

127 Giorgi 2016. Giorgi's main focus is the Byzantine aqueduct system, but she still focuses on the important Roman aqueduct there. Her assertion that the study of an aqueduct is crucial for understanding the daily life of a city is still valid for the discussion of Roman period water systems.

128 Grewe (2016) does offer a substantial synthesis of aqueducts in German, which is handsomely illustrated; however, it is crucial to produce an even greater study in English, using all available evidence. It should be noted that Camp (1991) already made the case for understanding the historical contexts of water supplies through diachronic and regional approaches.

of Roman bathing complexes, terminology, public and private baths, healing bathing complexes, and the cultural phenomena surrounding baths.[129]

Over the last few decades, the Greek precursors to Roman baths have become better understood by scholars, largely due to a number of archaeological discoveries that expanded the corpus of pre-Roman bathing complexes, definitely demonstrating that baths were built throughout the Greek world (including Egypt) well before Roman conquest.[130] Building upon the seminal work of Réné Ginouvès (1962), scholars have demonstrated how Greek bath structures started in the second half of the fifth century BCE and flourished in the Hellenistic period, with at least 75 known public baths, 17 baths connected to sports facilities (*gymnasia*/*palaestrae*), domestic baths, and others—more than half of which were unknown to Ginouvès.[131] The main purpose of the Greek bath structure was to provide a space for users to cleanse themselves. Public baths (*balaneia*) contained hip-bathtubs (made out of masonry or terracotta) that allowed individuals to wash themselves while seated, in addition to *louteria* (pedestal basins) that allowed for cleansing while standing; baths are characterized by at least one or two rooms, one of which is often circular to allow for a maximum number of hip-bathtubs that would have flanked the walls of the room.[132]

While Greek-style baths probably started in Athens in the late fifth century, they spread throughout the Greek world, including Magna Graecia in the late

129 Unlike other sections in the present discussion, the goal here is to highlight the recent developments in scholarship—understanding how the study of Roman baths has changed over the last three decades. See Manderscheid (2004) for a synthesis of bath bibliography up to the year 2001.

130 On Egypt, for example, see Boussac, Fournet, and Redon (2009), Fournet and Redon (2013), and Lucore (2016, 335–37), along with the French Balnéorient Project (http://balneorient.hypotheses.org, Last accessed 10 September 2017), which strives to publicize bath discoveries in Egypt.

131 Ginouvès' 1962 monograph was the first catalogue and synthesis of the available evidence of Greek bathing. There have been a few other studies since, but the most comprehensive (with bibliography) can be found in the conference proceedings, *Greek Baths and Bathing Culture: New Discoveries and Approaches*, by Sandra Lucore and Monika Trümper (2013), which brings together a variety of scholars to discuss numerous aspects of Greek bathing culture, culminating in a catalogue of 70 known Greek baths (identified by their inclusion of hip-bathtubs). Trümper's introduction provides a succinct state-of-the-field essay about Greek baths. Not included in the volume, however, was Wassenhoven's 2012 catalogue of baths of the Greek Peloponnese during classical antiquity. See also Yegül's discussion of Greek *gymnasia* and baths (1992, 6–29).

132 Lucore 2016, 330–31.

fourth century and Egypt in the Hellenistic period.[133] In Sicily and South Italy, experimental bathing technologies are found in bath complexes, including the earliest examples of furnaces (to allow for heated water) and hypocausts (to allow for immersion pools).[134] Indeed, by the Hellenistic period (mid-late fourth century BCE), Greek baths contained spaces intended for relaxing bathing—the prominent feature of Roman baths, which probably originated in the use of natural thermal waters in Sicily and Italy.[135]

The development and presence of heated baths in Sicily and South Italy has prompted much discussion about the transition from Greek-style bath complexes to their more distinct Roman counterparts. One of the earliest known examples of a Roman bath is the second building phase of a bath at Fregellae, a Latin colony in Latium, which dates to the second century BCE.[136] In this example, there are separate spaces for men and women,[137] rational organization of space, a large central furnace, a hypocaust system, and *alvei* (communal heated pools). The hypocaust system allows for heat to circulate beneath the floor, which is elevated by a series of small pillars made of square or circular bricks. The bath at Fregellae is one of the earliest known examples of this phenomenon. The organization of the space into a rational order, perhaps influenced by other examples on the Italian Peninsula, led to the tripartite division of early Roman baths: *apodyterium* (changing room), *tepidarium* (warm room), and *caldarium* (hot room).[138]

Fikret Yegül has spent much of his career exploring the development of Roman baths throughout the Roman world. He has shown that Roman bath complexes were a natural progression of Greek and native Italic models. Early Italian baths were often located near kitchens in domestic spaces, in order to take advantage of the already present heat sources, while also providing a space that allowed for healthy sweating (and probably later developed into the *laconicum*, or room intended for a dry heat, as opposed to the *sudatorium*,

---

133 Lucore 2016, 330–35.

134 Lucore 2016, 331–34. See especially Lucore's work on the baths of Morgantina in Sicily (e.g., Lucore 2013). For more on water management in Greek baths, see Manderscheid (2000a, 469–84).

135 Lucore 2016, 333.

136 Tsiolis (2013) and Yegül (2013).

137 Much has been written on gender issues in Greek and Roman baths. See Stähli (2013), who re-examines Greek vases that depict female bathers, suggesting that they may not be wholly accurate. For Roman baths, which seem to have been gender segregated early on and perhaps shifted in the Imperial period, see: Fagan (1999, 24–9) and Yegül (2010, 27–34).

138 Tsiolis 2013, 104–108.

for steamy heat).[139] The early development of Roman baths is easy to discern in the Bay of Naples region, with its well-preserved bath complexes, such as the Stabian Baths at Pompeii. In the second and first centuries BCE, in conjunction with newly developed technological advances in heating, the canonical 'single-axis row type' of Roman bath, which prompted patrons to progress from warm to hot rooms, from the *tepidarium* (warm room) to *caldarium* (hot room), in addition to the sweating rooms, often culminated in a plunge in the cold water pools of the *frigidarium*.[140] This particular bathing arrangement quickly spread beyond the Bay of Naples, and it can be seen throughout the Roman world.[141] Other spatial arrangements developed over time, including the 'half-axial type' (series of rooms that do not follow a strict axis of progression) and the symmetrical imperial baths of Rome (the series of rooms were replicated on a main central axis that provided bi-lateral symmetry).[142] There has been much scholarship on Roman baths outside of the Italian Peninsula, demonstrating the popularity of this cultural activity for nearly all the inhabitants of the empire.[143]

Roman bathing facilities naturally came in a variety of shapes and sizes, evident in the terminology the Romans themselves used for these spaces. In written sources, baths are known either as *balnea* or *thermae*.[144] The term *balnea* usually refers to smaller bathing establishments, such as a domestic bath suite or a neighborhood bath complex, the latter of which often had a nominal entrance fee;[145] while *thermae* was used to indicate the large-scale

139 Yegül 1992, 50–7; Yegül 2010, 45–7. Yegül (2010) is an update of his 1992 monograph, focusing primarily on Roman baths, using new scholarship and discoveries, while providing easily approachable syntheses of Roman bathing culture. See also the concise article of Fagan (2001) on the genesis of the Roman public bath.

140 Yegül 1992, 57–66; Gros 1996, 391–94; Yegül 2010, 51–8. On the bathing order of Roman baths, see Yegül (2010, 17–18).

141 Yegül 1992, 66–79; Yegül 2010, 58–65.

142 Yegül 1992, 80–91.

143 On North Africa, see: Yegül 1992, 128–183; Gros 1996, 409–13; Thébert 2003; Boussac, Fournet, and Redon 2009 (various essays on baths in Egypt); Yegül 2010, 133–53. On Asia Minor, see: Yegül 1992, 184–249; Farrington 1995 (on the region of Lycia); Gros 1996, 413–15; Yegül 2010, 154–80. On the provinces north of the Italian Peninsula, see: Gros 1996, 406–408. For relevant bibliography of archaeological discoveries of individual bath complexes throughout the empire until 2001, see Manderscheid (2004, 33–133). In Asia Minor, some large-scale façades in bath complexes have been associated with the imperial cult; see Burrell (2006, especially 450–53) for a pointed critique of these assumptions.

144 For more, see Fagan 1999, 14–9. See also Blonski 2014, 171–240.

145 Private domestic bath structures have been explored in-depth by Nathalie de Haan (2010), using evidence from the Italian Peninsula and North Africa, in order to explore not only

imperial bath complexes found both in Rome and abroad. The city of Rome at the end of the first century BCE had 200 *balnea*, but by the end of the fourth century CE, it is reported that *balnea* numbered at least 856, along with 10 or 11 *thermae*.[146] While the *balnea* were probably based on the 'single-row axis' or 'half-axis' types of arrangements, the imperial *thermae* often followed symmetrical arrangements. For example, the Baths of Caracalla in Rome have a strong axis of the *frigidarium-tepidarium-caldarium*, while there are two *palestrae* on opposite sides of the axis.[147] The *thermae* of Rome, provided by imperial benefaction (and thus with free entrance), were grand complexes that provided places for bathing, exercise, entertainment, and even eating and drinking. Among the most well known imperial *thermae* in Rome were those of Agrippa, Nero, Titus, Trajan, Caracalla, and Diocletian.[148] The Baths of Diocletian were the largest, and since it was later converted into the Church of Santa Maria degli Angeli, modern visitors can still gain a sense of its original grandiose scale. Due to the grandeur of these public complexes, some have interpreted imperial baths as 'palaces of the people,' where all inhabitants had access to the same services, thus underlining bathing facilities as important cultural and social institutions within the fabric of everyday Roman life.[149]

The remains of the Baths of Caracalla are still standing and have been relatively well studied, thereby offering a good example of the scale and costs of these monumental structures.[150] The complex consists of a main bathing core, which is surrounded by a precinct that provided libraries, meeting spaces (e.g., various types of performances), porticoes, water-displays, and shops (especially

their archaeological contexts but also their social implications. See Uytterhoeven (2012) for further bibliography and a brief discussion of private baths in the Roman East.

146 Yegül 2010, 2–3. The fourth-century numbers are derived from the *Notitia urbis regionum* (ca. 334–357 CE) and the *Curiosum urbis Romae* (357–403 CE).

147 On the symmetry of the imperial *thermae*, see Yegül (2010, 104).

148 For general discussions of these baths, see Yegül (1992, 128–83) and Yegül (2010, 101–32).

149 Scholarship has debated the inclusivity of Roman baths. It is generally agreed that while social barriers were not changed through bath access, there was indeed a mixing of different classes that was unique in the Roman social landscape. For more, see Yegül (2010, 34–39). Natascha Zajac (1999) argues that the grand imperial *thermae* of Rome were not built to improve the public health of the city's inhabitants, but were solely for the legitimization of the emperor.

150 On the Baths of Caracalla, see: Confronto 1991; Manderscheid 1991; DeLaine 1997; Jenewein 2008; Piranomonte 2012; Oetelaar 2013; Gensheimer forthcoming.

for foodstuffs).[151] The precinct itself measures nearly 1.3 km^2.[152] While the baths themselves are not innovative in terms of technology or construction technique, it is the actual scale of construction (some walls still survive to nearly 37 m high) and richness of decoration (e.g., imported marble and statuary) that make this complex especially impressive.[153] Through a careful architectural analysis, Janet DeLaine has posited that the baths would have cost nearly 12–14 million *kastrenses modii* (KM), broken down into materials (53% of the costs), decoration (29%), and amenities (17%), over the course of six or seven years for its construction.[154]

Roman bath technologies have also figured prominently in modern scholarship. Vitruvius in Book 5 of his treatise on architecture provides a brief discussion of necesssary factors in planning the construction of a bath complex, noting the features that make Roman baths unique from their predecessors, such as the hypocaust system (*De arch.* 5.10). The heating systems of baths included floor heating (the hypocaust), wall heating (including special tiles that allowed hot air to rise from the open cavities of the floors, the so-called nipple tiles (*tegulae mammatae*) and box-tiles (*tubuli*)), furnaces, *testidines alveolorum* (metal containers to keep water warm), and sweat rooms.[155] Water supply systems in baths were also intricately planned, as Hubertus Manderscheid has pointed out:[156] water had to be provisioned from a source, used, and then disposed of through drainage systems. Water actually had a number of functions within a bath complex: for primary facilities (namely cold water pools, hot water spaces, drinking water, and latrines, in addition to supplying *thermopolia*, watermills, and bakeries) and secondary uses (cleaning, watering plants, and decorative fountains).[157]

---

151 For more on the activities that took place in the *thermae*, see Yegül (2010, 119–32).

152 Piranomonte 2012, 10.

153 See especially DeLaine (1997, 9).

154 DeLaine 1997, 207–24, especially 219; for more on the design, decoration, materials, and construction process of the baths, see 45–194. DeLaine used the KM, which valued 100 *denarii* of wheat at 1 KM, in the *Price Edict* of Diocletian. The annual *annona* for 175,000 residents of Rome was valued at 7 million KM, the army annually cost the state between 44–150 million KM, and civilian salaries in Rome were between 4–6 million KM.

155 Yegül 2010, 80–97. See also Lehar (2012).

156 Manderscheid 2000a, 484–535. See also Yegül 2010, 97–100. Manderscheid also distinguishes between normal bathing facilities that only use fresh water, and those that use thermal and fresh waters, the latter of which would have different uses for the two types of water (see 511–14).

157 Manderscheid 2000a, 492–505.

Specific technical innovations have also seen an increased interest in modern scholarship. There have been a number of different experiments by scholars to understand exactly how floor and wall heating systems actually functioned.[158] In 1998, this type of experimentation was brought to a popular audience, when a team of scholars and specialists, led by Yegül, reconstructed a fully functioning Roman bath at Sardis, Turkey, which was sponsored by the television series *NOVA*.[159] The team's goal was to reconstruct a whole bath complex, including the thermal mechanisms of the heating system. Other interdisciplinary approaches to the archaeological evidence have employed modern engineering models to understand better how Roman baths functioned. For example, Ismini Miliaresis has studied the Terme del Foro of Ostia in terms of the fuel required for operating the baths. She has determined that 150 trees would need to be harvested, transported, and stored for the baths to run efficiently for an entire year.[160] Future studies in this same vein will surely yield better understandings of the complexities of Roman bathing complexes.

Roman baths are also found attached to naturally occurring thermal waters, which were prized for their healing qualities. Roman authors report on the medicinal and healing properties of these special waters, which probably increased their popularity.[161] Oftentimes known as spas (sometimes attributed to an abbreviation of *sanitas per aquam*, 'health through water'), bathing sites connected to healing waters were popular throughout the Roman Empire, such as Baiae in the Bay of Naples or Bath (Aquae Sulis) in England.[162] There were hundreds of healing spots, and many of these sites are still used today, preventing full archaeological investigation.[163] Indeed, many of these sites were simply called *Aquae* with an added qualifier (to differentiate one *Aquae* from the others), such as the locality's name, the site's founder, its divine connections, and/or a *cognomen*.[164] Some sites have been known for centuries,

158 For the complete bibliography, see Yegül and Couch (2003, 154, note 5).

159 Yegül and Couch 2003.

160 Miliaresis 2013. See also the earlier work of Blyth (1999).

161 Vitr. *De arch.* 8.3.1–5; Sen. *QNat* 3.2.1–2, 3.24; Pliny *NH* 31.1–2, 31.3.17, 31.32, 31.33–37. See Jackson (1999) for a succinct overview of ancient medical opinions regarding the healing properties of water; Fagan (1999, 85–103) offers the fullest discussion of medicinal waters in baths to-date, along with supplemental material from Köhler (2016).

162 On Baiae, see: Yegül 1992, 93–112; Yegül 1996; Nieberle 2016. On Bath, see: Cunliffe 1995; Revell 2009, 118–29. See also Donahue (2015) for a discussion of healing spas in Latium and Etruria.

163 Yegül 1992, 92.

164 For more on the phenomenon of *Aquae* throughout the empire, see Peréx and Rodríguez Morales (2011); Campbell (2012, 330–68). These types of healing sites are becoming

but have only recently undergone systematic excavations, such as Aquae Apollinares Novae (Vicarello, Italy) on Lake Bracciano, north of Rome.[165] The Domitianic era complex includes a bathing facility tied to the local thermal water that could reach up to 50 degrees Celsius, as well as an adjacent hostel, offering pilgrims a convenient way of extending their stay at the facilities. Indeed, spas were often built in scenic locations, with a number of amenities, so that patrons could not only heal their bodies and minds, but also enjoy a 'resort-like' space.[166] The hydrotherapeutic services of the spas could include both external and internal uses of water, such as full-body immersions or medicinal drinking water.[167] The sheer popularity of thermal bath complexes in the Roman world is easy to understand, as these types of health treatments are still popular today throughout the world.

In addition to archaeological evidence, Roman literature offers insight into Roman attitudes towards bathing culture. Seneca satirically bemoans many aspects of the baths, including the racket of rowdy bathers, which he suffered while living above a bath complex (*Ep.* 56) and the frivolous luxuries of contemporary baths compared to the Spartan example of Scipio Africanus (*Ep.* 86). While these passages cannot be taken at face value, they are helpful in reconstructing what types of activities and behaviors may have taken place in bath complexes, which is not immediately evident in the archaeological record. Garrett Fagan's 1999 monograph, *Bathing in Public in the Roman World*, is an invaluable resource, as it synthesizes literary, epigraphic, and archaeological sources to present a greater understanding of bathing in the Roman Empire, such as the popularity of the baths and the phenomenon of bath benefaction.[168] Another interesting avenue of inquiry that Fagan briefly explores is the notion of hygiene in the context of public baths. While Roman baths certainly improved the hygiene of the bathers, literary and epigraphic evidence suggest that baths could be dirty places, as some bathers did not take care to leave the space clean for other patrons.[169]

---

better published and known, such as those of the province of Hispania; see, for example, González Soutelo (2012). For a broad discussion of these types of healing sites, including their divine connections to Apollo, Asclepius, and the nymphs, see Rogers (2015, 331–51).

165 On the site at Vicarello, see Von Falkenstein-Wirth (2011).

166 Yegül 1992, 92–127; Köhler 2012.

167 Jackson 1999, 110–16.

168 Fagan's conclusions then inform other scholars, such as Yegül's brief synthesis of Roman bathing rituals and customs (2010, 11–21). See also Busch (1999), which is a similar treatment of the materials Fagan analyzed in German.

169 Fagan 1999, 181–88. Today's notions of hygiene, naturally stem from modern, post-Victorian conceptions of cleanliness that were not familiar to the ancients. For more on this concept, see Koloski-Ostrow (2015b, 102–104) and below, 39–46, on sanitation.

In the last few decades, a number of conferences on Roman baths have brought together new evidence from across large parts of the Roman world. The "First International Conference on Roman Baths," held in 1992 in Bath, England, organized by DeLaine and David Johnson, was divided into two parts: "Bathing and Society" explored bathing culture throughout different parts of the empire; while "Design and Concept" illustrated the need for further architectural studies and reconstructions of baths in various contexts (including around the Bay of Naples, military installations, and urban spaces)—a trend which has continued today in scholarship. The Frontinus Gesellschaft, in addition to the relevant bath entries in its *Cura Aquarum* series, organized a conference in Aachen in 2009 on the technical and cultural histories of Roman baths (*SPA: Sanitas per Aquam*).[170] The conference was able to pull together a wide variety of scholars who presented evidence from Italy, Greece, Turkey, Spain, Germany, Egypt, and elsewhere, thereby highlighting the many newly discovered and published sites (as well as some freshly re-examined cases) from throughout the Roman world.

Another significant research trend is the contextualization of Roman baths within the *longue durée* evolution of bathing practices extending to the present day. The beginning of this section focused on pre-Roman bathing facilities in the Greek world, demonstrating that the Roman bath was not *sui generis*; however, the technological advances of Roman baths, especially in terms of heating capabilities and water supply, were instrumental in providing a model for later bathing cultures. Yegül presents a succinct progression of baths from the Roman period into the Byzantine era, followed by a decline in bathing among Christians in the West and continued development under Islamic rule in the East.[171] Finally, he explores the development of modern notions of cleanliness and the importance of hygienic bathing in modern European societies, perhaps arising from the renaissance of 'oriental-style' bathing in the eighteenth and nineteenth centuries.[172]

4.4 *Drainage and Sanitation*

In the last twenty years, Roman drainage and sanitation have received a great deal of attention in modern scholarship. This research, employing new approaches and evidence, explores the systems themselves, frequently challenging modern notions about the cultural practices of the Romans. Following

170 Kreiner and Letzner 2012.

171 Yegül 2010, 181–212.

172 Yegül 2010, 213–30.

an overview of Roman drains and sewers, this section will present the relatively recent exploration of the Roman toilet, and then conclude by discussing the social implications of Roman sanitation practices and toilet usage, and how Romans conceptualized privacy and hygiene. Scholarship shows that the Roman world was indeed not as clean as modern audiences have come to believe.

Roman sewers and drains are of integral importance in dealing with water systems. In modern English, 'drains' refer to conduits that prevent impermeable surfaces, such as streets, from flooding; while 'sewers' traditionally refers to conduits used for human waste.[173] In Latin, however, it appears that no such distinction was made: *cloaca* (perhaps derived from *cluere*, to purge or to clean with running water) can signify a drain or sewer.[174] Given the wide regional variation in water management and technology, it is no surprise that different types of drainage systems were employed throughout the Roman world: open and closed drains, integrated drains (with both human waste and rainwater), and separated drain systems (one for waste and one for rainwater).[175] For the most part, it seems that Roman drains were 'conflated sewers,' in that they were intended to carry away excess waters in urban environments, but human sewage could also be present.[176] For clarity, scholars often divide drainage systems into four categories: first order (drains in a structure or complex, which leads waste away, e.g., gutters on roofs or channels from latrines); second order (combined first order drains to form a 'single exit channel'); third order ('principal canalizations,' which are generally underneath streets); fourth order (the collection of drains that discharge away from the settlement).[177] These four categories usually build upon each other to create an extensive urban drainage network that works effectively to move surplus water and human waste away from inhabitation.

The variety of drainage systems employed by the Romans is well documented in a 2000 article by Gemma Jansen. Using the archaeological evidence from Pompeii, Herculaneum, and Ostia, Jansen shows how local topography

173 Hodge 2002, 332; Koloski-Osüow 2015a, 80–2.

174 Reimers 1989, 137–38. Reimers also points out that the terms *fossa* and *cuniculus* could be used to indicate channels or trenches, such as agricultural drainage canals. Vitruvius also mentions that architects must be acquainted with the legal regulations surrounding drains, the *iura cloacarum* (*De arch.* 1.1.10). For more see Koloski-Ostrow (2015a, 63).

175 Reimers 1991, 112. For a more systematic treatment of these drain types, see Hodge (2002, 332–45) and Riera (1994, 399–415).

176 Koloski-Ostrow 2015a, 83.

177 Tölle-Kastenbein 1990, 170; Riera 1994, 399–415; Wilson 2000a, 152.

determines the type of conduit system a community could use. For example, because of Pompeii's steep gradient, rainwater could flow through the city and wash out at the lower city gates. In addition, Pompeii's low water table allowed for cesspits for private latrines, eliminating the need for an extensive sewer network.[178] Cesspits are holes in the ground that are dug to allow for the disposal of human waste. They act as liquid soak-aways, in that the liquid from the waste is allowed to soak down into the soil, while solid waste is left on top (and can be compacted), and later removed by *stercorarii*, the human waste collectors who would use the waste as agricultural fertilizer.[179] Given Herculaneum's steeper slope and harder volcanic soil, there are very few cesspits and limited sewers, as rain and wastewater could run off directly into the sea.[180] At Ostia, given the lack of gradient and high water table (especially with the proximity of the Tiber River), a large sewer network was installed to ensure proper waste management, as cesspits were impossible to use.[181] Thus, topography dictated exactly what type of drainage system a settlement could use.

Roman drains were built first and foremost to deal with wastewater. Frontinus even mentions that one of the main reasons for a drainage system, especially in Rome, was to deal with the water continuously running off from water fountains—and thus into the streets themselves (*Aq.* 111.2).[182] Indeed, in addition to flowing through streets, wastewater was important in all aspects

178 Jansen 2000b, 38.

179 For more on cesspits, see: Hodge (2002, 336–37), Jansen (2000b, 38), and Wilson (2000a, 175). For more on the *stercorarii*, see Wilson (2000a, 175–76).

180 Jansen 2000b, 43. For an updated in-depth investigation of the water supply and drainage systems of Herculaneum, see Camardo, Martelli Castaldi, and Thompson (2006), which is derived from the work of the Herculaneum Conservation Project begun in 2001.

181 Jansen 2000b, 45.

182 In modern scholarship, there have been questions regarding how much fountains could wash into the streets. In the case of small street fountains in Pompeii, for example, while occasionally they could flood the street with a limited amount of water, in reality, they probably only wetted the surrounding area of the street (Richard 2012, 130–31). There is a good amount of evidence from throughout the empire that excess water from fountains (especially large-scale examples) could go to secondary structures, such as latrines, before evacuating into drains (Richard 2012, 131, 135–36). There is no available evidence that public fountains could be switched off, using a stopcock, unlike private fountains (Richard 2012, 106). Richard, however, has recently demonstrated that the Late Hadrianic Nymphaeum at Sagalassos had a stopper on the parapet of its main basin, which would have prevented water run-off (Richard 2016a, 278–80). More research, it seems, needs to be conducted to understand better the potential to close off public fountains. For more on the ability for domestic fountains to be turned off, see Jansen (2001). For more on literary sources related to water control, see Reimers (1989) and Koloski-Ostrow (2015a, 63–5).

of Roman drainage. For example, surplus water from baths could be used to supply and clean out nearby latrines, and waste from sewers could be fed into fields as fertilizer.[183] Again, this reinforces the idea that Roman waste conduits functioned as 'conflated sewers.'[184]

Arguably the most famous drain in the Roman world was the Cloaca Maxima of Rome. The Great Drain was originally a small tributary of the Tiber River (with a zig-zagging course that led to the Tiber), which was reportedly canalized in the seventh century BCE by Tarquinius Priscus, as an open drain.[185] By the fifth century, the drain was monumentalized with lined stones, and was covered over in the late Republic. In the aedileship of Agripa in 33 BCE, a new lower stone course was added, monumentalizing it further. In past scholarship, the Great Drain has been associated with a great sanitary revolution in the city of Rome; however, recently, scholars have challenged that notion. In examining the physical remains of the Cloaca Maxima, Koloski-Ostrow believes that the structure was intended mainly as a storm drain, which could also serve other materials that entered it.[186]

Another crucial element of sanitation is the Roman toilet. While toilets have been identified since their excavation, it is only in the last few decades that they have received systematic attention by archaeologists.[187] The first major study of toilets was by Richard Neudecker (1994), which explores more luxurious toilets (the so-called *Prachtlatrine*) in the cities of the first two centuries of the Roman Empire. The studies of Barry Hobson (2009) expanded the

183 Wilson 2000a, 177. See also Hodges (2002, 335–36). For more on the use human excrement and urine, see Jansen, Koloski-Ostrow, and Moormann (2011b, 147–56) and Koloski-Ostrow (2015a, 89–92). Miko Flohr, an expert on *fullonicae*, or fulleries (spaces dedicated to the maintenance of wool fabrics), questions the old assumption that urine collection points were located outside *fullonicae* (e.g., amphorae on street corners), as this method of collection would ineveitably become contaminated. Evidently there must have been some other way that the *fullonicae* collected urine for their industrial uses. For more see Flohr (2011, 151–53).

184 Dion. Hal. *Ant. Rom.* 3.67.4–5. Koloski-Ostrow 2015a, 83.

185 For the previous bibliography of the Cloaca Maxima, see Gowers (1995) and Koloski-Ostrow (2015a, 63, note 66; 70, note 96), along with Hopkins on the early construction (2007) and on the drain's 'sacred' nature (2012). See also the collected volume of Bianchi (2015), which presents recent archaeological work done on the drain by the Sovrintendenza Capitolina ai Beni Culturali of Rome.

186 Koloski-Ostrow 2015a, 63–70, especially 70. Hopkins (2007) also makes this argument.

187 See more on the history of sanitation in Jansen, Koloski-Ostrow, Moorman (2011a, 2–3). In early excavations, toilets were not often identified as such (e.g., the machine chamber of a hydraulic lift).

discussion of toilets throughout the Roman world, offering a broader overview on the subject.[188] In 2007, the "Ancient Roman Toilet Workshop" was convened at the Royal Dutch Institute in Rome, bringing together an array of international scholars who work on Roman toilets, along with scholars of toilets from other time periods.[189] The resulting publication, *Roman Toilets: Their Archaeology and Cultural History*, is an important exploration of the cultural and social implications of toilets, their typology and placement in urban sanitation networks, and Roman styles of urination and defecation. One important contribution of the conference outlined regional trends in toilet usage across the Roman world, which might be based on cultural attitudes: more widespread use of toilets in the Italian Peninsula and North Africa, and less use of toilets in Britain, Syria, and Judea.[190]

The most recent monograph on Roman toilets, by Koloski-Ostrow (2015), offers an interdisciplinary study of Roman sanitation, using archaeological, literary, and epigraphic evidence from the Italian Peninsula (second century BCE to the second century CE).[191] While not a corpus of Roman toilets, Koloski-Ostrow's monograph is based on research conducted over the course of decades—its thoroughness illustrates some salient points about the subject. After a brief discussion of terminology (e.g., *latrina, secessus, necessaria, forica*),[192] Koloski-Ostrow delves into a wide body of evidence on the Italian Peninsula, proposes a latrine typology for the first centuries BCE and CE,[193] and demonstrates that Roman toilet forms were influenced by earlier precursors in the Hellenistic East.[194] In her discussion of Roman toilet use, Koloski-Ostrow engages the graffiti and paintings found in and around toilets, which

188 Hobson (2009b) explores the toilets of Pompeii, including those on second stories; Hobson (2009a) presents toilets from throughout the Roman world, with an emphasis on those found in Pompeii.

189 For more on the structure of the workshop, see Jansen, Koloski-Ostrow, Moorman (2011a, 3–5).

190 Jansen, Koloski-Ostrow, and Moormann 2011b, 183–87.

191 See Rogers (2016) for a short review of the monograph, which points out some of the very few problems with the study.

192 Koloski-Ostrow 2015a, 40–41. Oftentimes in modern scholarship, a distinction is made between a private toilet and public toilets (the multi-seater toilets), the latter of which is often described as a 'latrine.' See Jansen, Koloski-Ostrow, and Moormann (2011a, 4–5; 2011b, 43–7).

193 Koloski-Ostrow 2015a, 26–32. See also various discussions in Jansen, Koloski-Ostrow, and Moormann (2011b, 51–55, 100–102, 113–30).

194 Koloski-Ostrow 2015a, 52–63. See also chapter 3 in Jansen, Koloski-Ostrow, and Moormann (2011b, 21–42), which explores earlier toilets in Egypt, Jerusalem, and Greece.

often made jokes about defecation, but also issued warnings to those using latrines against those around them and the things lurking inside the toilets themselves.[195] Of particular interest in this study is the use of comparanda from other cultures regarding defecation, such as post-antique Europe, the Middle East, and Asia.[196]

The main achievement of Koloski-Ostrow's monograph is revisiting questions about Roman hygiene. It is often believed that the Roman world was a relatively clean place, given the presence of baths and drainage in most urban centers. This notion was first challenged by Alex Scobie in 1986, who also began engaging with the archaeological evidence of latrines and sewers, which were until then often neglected. By the late 1990s, more scholars were paying attention to this archaeological evidence, culminating in Günther Thüry's 2001 book on dirt in the Roman world and a conference in 1996 ("*Sordes Urbis*") about waste management in Roman cities.[197] Meanwhile, Garrett Fagan questioned the salubrious nature of Roman baths, especially given that the pools were used by healthy and sick alike, the waters changed probably only once a day, and the whole complex was likely saturated with γλοιός (a mixture of oil, sweat, and dirt, the by-product of strigiling one's body).[198] More recently, using comparative modern scientific data, the 2007 Roman Toilets Workshop further demonstrated that Roman latrines were indeed not hygienic according to modern standards. Toilet-related diseases could easily be transmitted in latrines because of how a Roman would clean him/herself after defecation (e.g.,

195 Koloski-Ostrow 2015a, 111–18; see also her discussion of Roman toilet use in Latin literature (104–11). See also on the images and graffiti associated with toilets, Jansen, Koloski-Ostrow, and Moormann (2011b, 165–81). Because Roman toilets and drain systems lacked traps, which close off the connection between the two, there was free movement of materials and organisms between the two. Thus, animals could appear in a toilet, having traveled from the drains themselves. For more, see Jansen, Koloski-Ostrow, and Moormann (2011b, 159) and Koloski-Ostrow (2015a, 82–83). Presumably, the fear associated with these creatures led to the worship of Fortuna in and around toilets, hoping that she would bring luck and protection, especially against the Evil Eye (Koloski-Ostrow 2015a, 113–14).

196 Koloski-Ostrow 2015a, 41–8.

197 Dupré Raventós and Remolà Vallverdú (2000) edited the "*Sordes Urbis*" conference proceedings, which has a wide range of essays, including some on rubbish disposal in the Roman city. Another more recent edited volume on waste management in the Iberian Peninsula can be found in Remolà Vallverdú (2011), along with the review by Koloski-Ostrow and Ostrow (2014). See also Cilliers (1993), who examines possible Roman state interest in public health through legal policies.

198 Fagan 1999, 176–88; Fagan 2000. See also the discussion in Jansen, Koloski-Ostrow, and Moormann (2011b, 158–59).

what was the role of washbasins?) and how domestic toilets (often connected to cesspits) were located adjacent to kitchens.[199] Koloski-Ostrow, picking up on this previous scholarship, makes the case that modern scholars must divorce themselves from modern standards of hygiene, which did not develop until the mid-nineteenth century, and evaluate the ancient evidence appropriately.[200]

The most recent research on Roman hygiene has focused on how toilets were actually *used* by ancient Romans. One persistent question about Roman toilet use is that of privacy. Public latrines, while usually multi-seaters, would nevertheless have offered some privacy, with offset doors (to prevent outsiders looking in) and high windows (to make the space dark). And although the seats were typically situated relatively close together, users presumably would have afforded themselves greater privacy by pulling the folds of their clothes around their genitals while seated.[201] It has been argued that the proliferation of public toilets (from the time of Augustus throughout the first two centuries CE) was part of the élite class' method of controlling social order, creating a confined space for behaviors that would otherwise have taken place out in the open.[202] Another question of toilet use is how the Romans cleaned themselves afterward. The perennial favorite of the 'sponge stick' (i.e., a sponge attached to a stick for self-cleaning) has found traction over the years, as it is mentioned a few times in Latin literature and occasionally sponge spicules are found in toilet drains.[203] In public latrines, conduits located in front of the seats, presumably filled with running water, have been interpreted as spaces to rinse sponge sticks. But there has been some resistance to the notion that sponge sticks were used in public latrines or that they were used communally (thereby exacerbating already questionable hygienic conditions). Lastly, scholars have recently posed questions about the sensory experience of using dark, not well-ventilated public latrines with drains that were not always

199 Jansen, Koloski-Ostrow, and Moormann 2011b, 157–64. On the evidence for washbasins, see Jansen, Koloski-Ostrow, and Moormann (2011b, 104–105). For more on the proximity of private toilets to kitchens, see Jansen, Koloski-Ostrow, and Moormann (2011b, 123–26).

200 Koloski-Ostrow 2015a, especially 118–22. See also Jansen (2000a).

201 Koloski-Ostrow 2015a, 92–6. For more on the notions of windows and lighting in public latrines, see Koloski-Ostrow 2015a, 28–9.

202 Koloski-Ostrow 2015a, 96–8. See also Jansen's 2003 study of the toilets of Hadrian's Villa at Tivoli. In her analysis she differentiates between the various toilets found there—and who potentially was able to use them (e.g., emperor; imperial retinue; slaves).

203 Jansen, Koloski-Ostrow, and Moorman 2011b, 102–104; Koloski-Ostrow 2015a, 86–8. Koloski-Ostrow supports the sponge stick theory, but does not address the counter arguments in her text.

continuously flushed.[204] While to the modern audience a Roman toilet might be unbearable, it is worth remembering that the ancients, accustomed to an environment of odors (which might be considered foul today), probably had a sensory landscape distinct from that of today.[205]

4.5 *Water-Displays*

The study of Roman water-displays has a rich and vibrant history, and one that is constantly evolving. Over the course of the last century, scholarship has moved away from strict typologies and catalogues, attempting to understand fountains in their original context of Roman society and the built environment. At this point, scholars are fortunate to be able to draw evidence from across the empire, in order to put together a 'bigger picture' of Roman water-display. Like other aspects of Roman water culture, water-displays come in public and private contexts, which can impact their usage and meaning for an ancient audience.

Before turning to the modern scholarship, however, the terminology of Roman water-displays must be discussed briefly. Romans had a veriety of at least 21 different terms for fountains, suggesting they themselves were fluid in word choice for their water-displays.[206] Of those terms, *nymphaeum* has come down through modern scholarship to refer occasionally to private fountains, while more often indicating the monumental fountains of the empire, such as the large water-displays seen in the city of Rome itself (e.g., the Severan Septizodium) or in Asia Minor, a region known for its large, showy fountains.[207] But the term 'nymphaeum' became popular only in the modern period—especially during the Renaissance, when it was used to describe fountains (often of a grotto-like appearance) in Italian villas.[208] And there are a few problems with this popular usage. First, the word has religious connotations, stemming

204 Jansen, Koloski-Ostrow, and Moormann 2011b, 181–83.

205 Koloski-Ostrow 2015b.

206 The terms include: *alveus, cantharus, castellum* [*aquae/divisorium*], *cisterna, concha, crater, euripus, hydreion/ὑδρεῖον, hydrekdocheion/ὑδρεκδοχεῖον, labrum, lacus, Meta Sudans, munus, nymphaeum/νυμφαῖον, phiala, puteus, saliens, septizodium, silanus*, and *solium*. The meaning of these terms is discussed in detail by Settis (1973), Letzner (2013), and Rogers (2015, 30–79; 2018, 173–74).

207 For more on the number and reasons for the large-scale fountains of Asia Minor, see the recent article of Lendon (2015), which posits that the influx of monumental fountains there after the Flavian period can be attributed to the formal education of young men, which included extolling the importance of water in urban settings.

208 Richard 2012, 2–4.

from the sacred spaces of nymphs, especially in the Greek world.[209] And yet, by the High Roman Empire, large-scale fountains had been divorced from this religious association, unlike natural springs, which might be the object of ritual and cult.[210] Indeed, in the Roman period, fountains were man-made structures built either *de novo* or over a natural water source.[211] Second, 'nymphaeum' in modern usage typically implies a certain level of monumentality. Modern scholarship often deems any large-scale fountain a 'nymphaeum,' even without epigraphic evidence that the ancients themselves called the structure a 'nymphaeum.'[212] Given the handful of inscriptions still remaining, it is difficult to apply 'nymphaeum' universally to all fountains.

Given the widespread adoption of 'nymphaeum,' the word also cannot simply be rejected. Other terms, however, can be employed to avoid this problem of anachronistic connotation, such as 'fountain' or 'water-display.' A water-display has two functions: to show off water and to collect the water for a secondary use, such as ritualistic washing or refreshment. A water-display, and by extension 'fountain,' then, is not restricted to a particular size, which means that a wider body of examples can be used in studying Roman fountains—not just the often impressive monumental façades that one associates with nymphaea.

Roman fountains came in many sizes and shapes, constantly evolving and adapting over time. Greek and Hellenistic fountains were generally tied directly to springs or simple aqueduct channels, and most were covered structures that prevented water from evaporating quickly, thereby aiding water conservation.[213] Under Augustus, especially with the growth of the water supply system under Agrippa, the city of Rome witnessed the advent of monumental fountains, whose architectural forms drew inspiration from Republican and early imperial domestic spaces.[214] What immediately distinguished Roman public fountains from their Greek counterparts was the

209 Walker 1979, 20–41; Walker 1987; Richard 2012, 4–7.

210 See below, 76–8, for more on the religious nature of water in the Roman world.

211 For example, see Agusta-Boularot (2001, 167–68) and Longfellow (2011, 9–13).

212 There are a handful of inscriptions that describe fountains as 'nymphaea' in the Roman world, including the first-century-CE *nymphaeum* from Metz, France (*CIL* 13.4325), the 104–105 CE Trajanic fountain in Syria (*Inscriptiones graecae ad res romanas pertinentes* 3.1273), and the second half of the second-century νυμφαῖον from the Agora of Argos (Argos Inv. E.266). For a complete discussion of the epigraphic evidence, see: Settis (1973).

213 Longfellow 2011, 9–13; Richard 2012, 34–40. Longfellow in particular traces the development of monumental Roman fountains from their Greek precursors through the third century CE.

214 Longfellow 2011, 3.

ostentatiously wasteful use of water, insofar as these displays were often uncovered, prioritizing public display over water conservation—a feat made possible due to the increase in reliable water supply. The construction of fountains continued in Rome through the Flavians, including the famed Flavian-period Meta Sudans, built on the foundations of an Augustan predecessor.[215] When the emperor Hadrian began traveling throughout the empire, he sponsored the construction of water-displays and water supply systems, especially in Greece and Asia Minor. In Greece, the water-displays were constructed using Italian architectural models (such as the semi-circular, open air nymphaeum in the Athenian Agora), as well as Greek models (such as the basilica-form nymphaeum on the slopes of the Larissa Hill at Argos).[216] In Turkey, Hadrian plugged into a pre-existing culture of aquatic benefactions sponsored by the local élite class, thereby producing the famous Baroque-style façade fountains found up and down the coast of Asia Minor.[217] Back in Rome, the Severans reintroduced the monumental fountain, including the famous Septizodium near the Circus Maximus, which included both features found previously in Rome and architectural innovations from the provinces.[218]

Naturally, not all Roman water-displays were 'monumental.' The streets of Roman cities throughout the empire were outfitted with fountains, providing easily accessible water for the local populations.[219] Most often, these were simple rectangular structures, built by joining four stone blocks in the form a basin, with a pillar providing the water that flowed into the basin.[220] The Romans called these fountains either a *lacus* or a *saliens*; the former indicates a hollow cavity, while the latter implies a structure with 'jumping' or 'gushing' water.[221] Water-displays were also attached to other architectural elements, thereby lending a sense of vitality to a structure. There are a number of such water-displays attached to arches and gates throughout the Roman Empire.[222] For example, the North Nymphaeum at the foot of Perge's acropolis was designed so that water flows through both an arch and a sculpture of a personified

215 Longfellow 2010; 2011, 3, 31–49.

216 Longfellow 2011, 120–31. See also Vitti (2016, 127–32) for more on the Argos nymphaeum, which challenges the reconstructions of Leigh (1998, 139) and Longfellow (2011, 113–20), based on a careful autopsy of the architectural present remains of the structure.

217 Longfellow 2011, 140–62.

218 Lusnia 2004; Longfellow 2011, 163–83.

219 Agusta-Boularot 2008.

220 Del Chicca 1997, 234.

221 Rogers 2015, 37–41, 60–3. For more on the differences between the *lacus* and *saliens*, see Del Chicca (1997) and Ambrogi (2005, 58).

222 Rogers 2015, 215–46.

local water source (the Kestros River), before continuing through the main thoroughfare of the city in a *euripus* (water channel).[223] Some theaters were also fitted with water-displays on the *frons pulpiti* (or front of the stage), which not only provided small displays of splashing water when theatrical productions were not taking place, but also cooled the surrounding air.[224] Within domestic spaces, at both urban and extra-urban locations, water-displays could come in a variety of forms, including water channels, aedicular structures with spouts in their interior niches, and dining spaces with water flowing around them.[225] Whatever the form or scale, water-displays were present throughout the Roman Empire in a variety of contexts, demonstrating the ubiquity of flowing water in the Roman world.

Modern scholarship includes general publications on fountains, typologies, catalogues based on geography, syntheses, connections with water networks, and empire-wide studies. First, there have been general archaeological publications of the various water-displays throughout the empire. Monographs such as Renate Bol's work on the Nymphaeum of Herodes Atticus in Olympia (1984) and Robinson's magisterial study of the Peirene fountain of Corinth (2011) have reexamined specific monuments, altering previous conceptions of those water-displays and their complex histories. Current and ongoing research projects by groups of scholars, especially the field reports found in the publications of the *Cura Aquarum* series, provide up-to-date excavation results and interpretations. Without the diligence of these field archaeologists, proper data would not be available to be mobilized within theoretical models.

Second, there is the great tradition of Roman water-display typologies. The two most important contributions are Neuerburg (1965) and Letzner (1990; 1999). Norman Neuerburg, studying the public and private water-displays of the Italian Peninsula, suggests that there are six different types of fountains (*edicola, camera, facciata, grotta, semicircolare*, and *rotondi*) and analyzes their placement within the greater context of their location. Wolfram Letzner illustrates 458 public and private water features in the western half of the Roman Empire. His extensive catalogue allowed him to offer a *Grobtypologie*, or a broad typology, of 19 variations of water features, thereby placing these water-displays in their wider typological context.[226] Hélène Dessales has recently built on the work of Neuerburg and Letzner, offering new typologies of

223 Dorl-Klingenschmid 2001, cat. no. 85; Longfellow 2011, 156–61; Aristodemou 2012, cat. nos. 234–242; Richard 2012, cat. no. 59; Rogers 2015, 227–30.

224 Rogers 2015, 377–88; 2018, 183–88.

225 Dessales 2013; Rogers 2013.

226 Letzner (1999) is a second revised edition of the 1990 original publication.

basins, fountain elevations, and fountain furniture (i.e., moveable objects associated with a water-dsiplay, including sculpture, vases, and miniature fountains), on the basis of finds from Pompeii and comparanda from other parts of the empire.[227] Other briefer studies present similar typological discussions, including those by S. Meschini (1963), Ginouvès (1969), Salvatore Settis (1973), and Pierre Aupert (1974).

Third, water-displays are organized into catalogues, which are typically grouped by region. The fountains of Italy are gathered in the extensive catalogue of Neuerburg, which includes both public and private examples. Understanding the site of Ostia was supplemented in 1996 by the study of Ricciardi and Scrinari. The western half of the empire, as already mentioned, was catalogued by Letzner. Knowledge of North African water-displays was improved with Francesco Tomasello's study of the minor fountains and nymphaea of Leptis Magna (2005) and Nicolas Lamare's recent dissertation (2014), which catalogues the monumental fountains of Northern Africa. The eastern half of the empire has likewise been covered by a series of regionally-based catalogues: Greece by Susan Walker (1979), Franz Glaser (1983), and Sandrine Agusta-Boularot (2001); Asia Minor by Claudia Dorl-Klingenschmid (2001); Asia Minor and the Middle East by Richard (2012; 2016b); the Middle East by Arthur Segal (1997).

Recently, the fountains of Roman Gaul have also received attention in secondary scholarship. Henri Lavagne, over the course of his career, has illustrated a number of Gallic water-displays (1990; 1992; 2012). Claude Bourgeois (1991; 1992a) has presented the evidence for both indigenous and Roman water cults, as well as their associated monuments, in the area of modern France. Agusta-Boularot, in her 1997 dissertation, outlines the development of water-displays throughout the empire, incorporating examples from France. In a 2004 issue of *Dossiers d'Archeologie*, edited by Agusta-Boularot, a number of French archaeologists present examples of fountains, including new reconstructions, from throughout Roman Gaul, making them accessible to a wider audience. Unfortunately, these Gallic examples are often left out of the 'canon' of Roman water-displays, perhaps due to issues in terminology and misunderstandings of local trends in fountains in France.[228]

227 Dessales 2013, 53–176. See a helpful critical review of Dessales' study by Keenan-Jones (2016).

228 Scholars note the difficulty in the appellation 'nymphaeum' to any water-display in France, which might have religious or monumental connotations (Bourgeois 1992a, 21; 1992b, 107–12; Lavagne 2012, 422). Lavagne himself wonders why more 'nymphaea' (i.e., what might be considered a 'monumental' fountain) in France are not given over to local

Work on domestic fountains has also become a vibrant field of study. Again, Neuerburg is the earliest collection of examples in Italy, which has since been supplemented by Ricciardi and Scrinari (1996) for Ostia, Marianna Bressan (2003) for examples throughout Italy (especially subterranean ones), and Dylan Rogers for Pompeii (2013). Mantha Zarmakoupi (2014), in her study of luxury villas on the Bay of Naples, provides an in-depth discussion of water in those structures, focusing on their meaning and architectural importance for those spaces. Zarmakoupi illustrates different types of water-displays, including nymphaea and *euripi*, and the spaces designated for swimming and sunbathing in a villa. She concludes that beyond the symbolic and mythological associations of flowing water, the water-displays were a fashionable demonstration of wealth and available luxury. Imperial villas have also received attention for their water-displays, especially Hadrian's Villa near Tibur (modern Tivoli).[229] The villa's abundance of water (nearly 300 discharge points for water!) vitalized the surrounding architecture and highlighted not only the power of the emperor (who had access to this water), but also his physical presence in the villa, as many of these water-displays directed one's view to the emperor himself. While the scale and complexity of water-displays might be different in an imperial villa versus a private villa or *domus*, in both contexts there was the desire and ability to show water off in a variety of ways.

Dessales' 2013 monograph most fully explores domestic fountains of Roman Italy, using examples from around the empire to supplement her arguments. In addition to offering a catalogue and typologies of fountain elements, Dessales places the fountains of Pompeii into their urban water network, demonstrating that private fountains at Pompeii (and probably elsewhere) were not used for drinking water, but rather for display and other secondary uses, such as for baths.[230] Because a Roman house probably had access to various types of water (rain, ground, and piped waters), drinking water evidently came from a

religious worship (1992, 224); however, he also states that fountains in Gaul often adopt Italian models (1990, 137; 2012, 138). Even Agusta-Boularot states that 'monumental' fountains were rare in France before the second century CE (2004, 7). There are a number of examples, however, of fountains in Roman Gaul that use both local and Roman styles of design and display of water that make France a unique and important point of dialogue on Roman water-displays.

229 The bibliography on Hadrian's villa is vast, but see the following for succinct discussions of the water-displays there: Ehrlich 1989; MacDonald and Pinto 1995; Salza Prina Ricotti 1998; Manderscheid 2000b, 2002, 2010. The recent collected volume of Fahlbusch (2008) examines the use of water of the villa, with emphasis on the water sources themselves.

230 Dessales 2013, 305–306, 317–31.

mixture of those sources, and the water flowing through fountains, although it could drain into a cistern for secondary use, was not intended for drinking.[231]

Dessales' work is particularly notable for its exploration of the placement of water-displays within the domestic sphere. Most attention to-date has been paid to the role of water in spaces associated with gardens in domestic structures.[232] For example, Wilhelmina Jashemski, the pioneering archaeologist who developed archaeological methods to uncover Roman gardens, vividly illustrates the use of water in Pompeian gardens: pools, fountains, sculpture, and mosaic fountains.[233] Studies of water-displays demonstrate the importance of the visibility of fountains through the entrances of Pompeian homes, reflecting the luxury and power of the owner as someone who could afford to display flowing water.[234] Dessales, however, shows that over time water infiltrated nearly every part of the Roman house (especially after the rise in available water from imperially-sponsored aqueducts), not just the peristyle where it traditionally appeared in houses throughout the Italian Peninsula.[235]

The proper discussion of the historical development of water-displays throughout the empire has been greatly facilitated by field reports, typologies, and catalogues. Pierre Gros (1996) offers one of the most succinct and well-informed discussions of how fountains transformed over time, with attention to different contexts throughout the whole empire. Dorl-Klingenschmid (2001) provides a diachronic narrative of how fountains changed in their urban contexts. Brenda Longfellow (2011) has recently examined the development of monumental fountains in Rome, Greece, and Asia Minor, attempting to place

231 See also Keenan-Jones 2016, 785.

232 Neuerburg 1965, 87–8.

233 Jashemski 1979, 32–49. The study of Roman gardens (and others in the ancient world) has been growing over the last decade, whether spurred on by Jashemski's archaeological work or in studies of the garden in Roman literature. For example, see Kathryn Gleason's edited volume, *A Cultural History of Gardens in Antiquity* (2013), Kathleen Coleman's edited volume, *Le jardin dans l'antiquitè* (2014), Farrar (1998; 2016), and, most recently, the long awaited volume by Jashemski et al. (2017). See Wescoat (2013) for an overview of waterworks in the study of garden archaeology worldwide.

234 Rogers 2013, 157–58.

235 Dessales 2013, 333–80. Dessales also discusses the development of the private water-display, stemming from Egypt, Magna Graecia, palaces in the East, and then Republican-era villas on the Italian Peninsula (2013, 13–51).

them in an empire-wide progression.[236] Lamare also provides a succinct overview of how water-displays throughout the empire developed.[237]

Next, public water-displays have recently been studied in terms of their placement in water infrastructure systems. De Kleijn, in her 2001 study of the water supply of Rome, illustrates how the larger water system of Rome impacted the numerous ways that water was used in the capital, and offers a series of water usage categories (recreational, personal, domestic, operational, and aesthetic). Richard (2007; 2012) stresses that water-displays must be studied in terms of their wider water systems, arguing that displays cannot be properly understood without knowing how water reached them or how much water might have been available. In a similar vein, Cecelia Weiss (2011) has recently highlighted the impact of geology on Roman water-displays, building upon Dora Crouch's work on Greek water supply and usage (1993; 2003).

Finally, the study of water-displays now seeks to place ancient Roman fountains into wider-reaching contexts throughout the empire, including aesthetic trends, urban contexts, social considerations, and little explored public contexts. In terms of aesthetics, the decoration of water features has been considered in different respects. Deena Berg (1994) explores the artistic development of fountains, from 700 to 30 BCE, providing a foundation for subsequent studies of Roman structures. The seminal work on Greek and Roman fountain sculpture is still that of Balázs Kapossy (1969). The sculptural programs of water-displays in the eastern half of the empire have also received greater attention in later studies, such as the monograph of Georgia Aristodemou (2012) and a few recent dissertations (e.g., Chi 2002; Ng 2007; and Taback 2002). Dorl-Klingschmid, in her 2001 study, classifies water-displays as *Prunkbrunnen* (decorative fountains), and gathers examples based on form, decoration, and placement within the cityscape.

Analyses of the urban contexts in which water-displays appear have provided fruitful results in the last two decades. Moving past simple typologies, scholars have studied fountains in their original contexts, understanding better how they function in urban spaces. The dissertation of Agusta-Boularot (1997) illustrates the importance that water-displays could have in Roman cities, particularly in the western half of the empire. S. Ellis (1997) argues for the use of water infrastructure (including aqueducts and fountains) as a means of social

236 Criticism of Longfellow's work has focused in particular on her data set, which examines only examples dedicated to the emperor (either by the emperor himself, imperial officials, or members of the local élite class). See Campagna (2011), Burrell (2012), and Lavagne (2012).

237 Lamare 2014, 1.93–127.

control in Rome and the provinces. Schmölder-Veit (2009) examines urban sites in Italy, North Africa, Spain, and Switzerland, investigating the relationship between fountains and the urban water supply. Nur Banu Uğurlu (2009) examines the placement of Roman fountains throughout Asia Minor; while Longfellow (2011) explores expressions of patronage and identity through water-displays, primarily using examples from this region. Finally, Richard (2012) has been at the forefront of interpreting water-displays in terms of identity and placing these structures in their original socio-economic, socio-cultural, and socio-political contexts.

Water-displays have been studied by scholars for their implications about Roman society and landscape, including their role as status symbols, products of patronage and munificence, and as indicators of identity.[238] Walker (1979) is an early example of placing large-scale fountains in their wider cultural milieu to illustrate how Greeks in the Roman period employed water-displays as markers of their social standing within their communities. Shaw (1991), focusing on North Africa, demonstrates the need for approaching water usage at the regional level. Here, Shaw shows the luxurious and utilitarian nature of water, along with the increasing desire of the local élite to use water in new fashionable ways. Wilson (1995) also explores the use of water in North Africa and shows that water throughout this large region was generally a marker of luxury and status, as some sites were not as well watered as those in the more northernly parts of the Mediterranean basin. Susanna Piras (2000) likewise demonstrates that water-displays could act as a powerful status symbols, especially those that featured water without any functional purpose or secondary use (although this was probably not the case with most fountains throughout the empire). Robinson (2013) suggests that the fountains of Corinth, many of which are tied to old Greek myths (e.g., Peirene was the site where Bellerophon tamed Pegasus), helped the new Roman inhabitants of the *colonia* forge a new identity, one uniquely Roman and Greek at the same time.

Another trend in recent studies has been to approach water-displays from the standpoint of religion and entertainment. New discoveries, naturally, continue to change the narrative of water-displays in these contexts, making the already rich corpus of fountains even more so. For example, a large three-terraced nymphaeum (perhaps dedicated to Egeria) from the Caligulan period was recently discovered at the Sanctuary of Diana at Nemus Aricinum (Nemi, Italy).[239] Constructed within a liminal space outside of the sanctuary proper,

238 See also the recent dissertation by Lytle (2015) for more on Republican and Early Augustan fountains in Rome (*non vidi*).

239 Braconi 2013; Rogers 2015, 309–12.

the large nymphaeum lavishly illustrated the flowing water of the natural source located there. Longfellow (2012) also demonstrates the power of Romans adding fountains to preexisting Greek religious sanctuaries in Greece in Asia Minor, showing that the Romans were able to make bold statements regarding their presence in the East, while at the same time expressing religious reverence in sites such as Eleusis, Olympia, and Xanthos. Rogers explores the use of water-displays in religious sanctuaries throughout the empire: source and healing sanctuaries in the west; fountains at sanctuary entrances in the East; and fountains connected to imperial cult buildings throughout the empire.[240] Further, more attention is being paid to water in Roman theaters, from the use of water on the *frons pulpiti*, its presence in the *porticus postscaenium*, the phenomenon of aquatic spectacles in and around orchestras, to the exchange of architectural vocabulary between theaters and fountain structures.[241] Thus, there are new ways that scholars can use new and already existing pieces of evidence to explore water-displays more fully.

Finally, phenomenological studies are beginning to explore how Romans themselves would have experienced their fountains. It is difficult, of course, to repopulate ancient spaces with bodies. Yet one can draw on comparative studies of more modern fountains and consider how interactions with water today may reflect the experiences of ancient Romans. Popular fascination with the Baroque Trevi Fountain in Rome has been explored by John Pinto (1986), tracing its meaning and power from its construction to the present day. Katherine Rinne in various publications has made the case for the visceral power of water and its special place in the fountains of Rome (1999; 2010). A 1998 exhibition at the Cooper-Hewitt National Design Museum in New York explored the spectacle and pleasure of fountains from the Renaissance to the modern period.[242] The work of Rogers examines Roman water-displays in terms of how the canonical five senses can effect and affect an ancient Roman's experience with a structure, regardless of context or location throughout the empire. In his 2015 dissertation, public fountains are explored in various contexts (civic, religious, and entertainment-related), illustrating that fountain placement, design, and water usage were similar throughout the empire, given humans' common and

240 Rogers 2015, 266–354.

241 See Rogers (2015, 355–406) for an in-depth discussion of these issues, see also Rogers (2018, 183–88), along with Day (2017). On the aquatic spectacles of the Roman theater, see: Traversari (1960); Berlan-Bajard (2006), which is reviewed by Coleman (2008). On the relationship between theater and fountain architecture, see Aristodemou (2011) and Lamare (2011). See also below, 70–5, for more on aquatic spectacles.

242 Symmes 1998.

innate sensory response to water. Further work by Rogers focuses on public and private examples in Roman Greece, with particular attention to sensory experiences.[243]

4.6 *Hydraulic Power*

Given the ubiquity of water in the Roman world, there were many uses that fit outside what one may consider the canonical uses of water—particularly in hydraulic-powered systems, which powered the Roman economy, both literally and figuratively. Throughout the ancient world were many different water-lifting devices in various forms.[244] They often served a variety of purposes: aiding agricultural irrigation;[245] facilitating work in mines; obtaining water from wells; assisting fire prevention. Some of the most prominent and efficient devices in the Roman world were the compartmental wheel and the water-screw, the chain pump, and force pumps. Devices in wheel forms are the most efficient lifting devices, as the force of the moving water actually moves the devices themselves.[246] The Roman force pump, which could be made from a variety of materials including wood, was based on Greek models, but simplified for ease of use.[247] Force pumps were probably also used in the Roman theater for liquid *spartiones*, which would have run down the *cavea*, spraying the surrounding air with scented and colored water.[248] While the Roman world was probably filled with a number of different water-lifting devices and technologies, only scant examples have survived since antiquity, making a complete study of them difficult.

Water was also used to power mills throughout the Roman world. Mills have been in continuous use since antiquity, and modern scholarship over time

243 Rogers 2018; Rogers forthcoming. Sensory studies are growing in modern studies on Greco-Roman culture. For the most recent collected volume of Betts on multisensory experiences in Roman culture (2017).

244 See Oleson (1984; 2000b) for a complete overview of Greek and Roman water-lifting devices, for which there were many. There is a great Hellenistic tradition of literature on water-lifting devices and other similar apparatuses that relied on hydraulics. For more see Lewis (2000).

245 For more on agricultural irrigation practices, see Oleson (2000a) and Wilson (2008, 309–10).

246 Oleson 2000b, 229.

247 The force pump sits in the water or liquid that it is moving, and thus is not a modern siphon pump. For more on the force pump itself, see: Oleson 2000b, 272–85; Fleury 2005; Brun and Fiches 2007; Fleury 2008a; Stein 2014.

248 Fleury 2008b. For more on the use of *spartiones* in the Roman theater, see Rogers (2015, 356–57; 2018, 183), along with Day (2017).

has debated their importance for various cultures in different time periods.[249] Currently, over 60 Roman mills are known.[250] There were different arrangements of wheels in mills: wheels could be vertical or horizontal; placed in a source of moving water, either natural bodies of waters (e.g., streams or rivers) or manmade open aqueduct channels.[251] On the Janiculum hill, a watermill, with five millraces, connected to the Aqua Traiana was partially excavated in the 1990s, perhaps illustrating the importance of these structures in the reorganization of the *annona* in the third century CE.[252] A large-scale example of a compound watermill is that of the complex found at Barbegal (7 km west of Arles, France), which lies on a steep gradient descending nearly 30 m.[253] The large building (61 × 20 m) was separated into a series of rooms; water flowed in through two main channels, powering seven wheels on either side, which ran the mill. The structure itself, because of its size and preservation, marks it as one of the most important flourmills in the Roman world, active from the first to third centuries CE.

Mills were not limited to simply grinding grain. There is evidence that watermills were used to power saws, such as the examples found at Hierapolis (Turkey) from the second half of the third-century and at Jerash (Jordan) from the late fifth-century.[254] Further, mills were used to power industrial mining activities, from prospecting and extracting, to primary ore-processing.[255] Scholars have noted that the mechanized technologies associated with watermills played a significant role in the growth of the Roman economy, from the first century CE on.[256] Wilson has argued that the cessation of water-related mining techniques in the third century CE adversely impacted the Roman economy, because easily mined gold and other metals could no longer contribute to the precious metal market economy.[257] Due to the paucity of evidence for mills, however, the field is still nascent.

249 Despite archaeological discoveries of ancient mills in the twentieth century, economic historians in the middle of the century attempted to deny the importance of these structures in antiquity. For more on this debate, see Greene (1994) and Wikander (2000, 371).

250 Wikander 2000, 372. See the relevant chapters in Brun and Fiches (2007) on mills.

251 Wikander 2000, 373, 378; Wilson 2002, 9–15.

252 Bell 1994; Wilson 2000c. See Taylor (2010) for more on the third-century reorganization of the *annona*.

253 Leveau 1996; 2007.

254 Wilson 2002, 16. On the Hierapolis example, see Ritti, Grewe, and Kessner (2007), and Seigne (2006) for the Jerash example.

255 Wilson 2002, 17–23.

256 Wilson 2002; Bruun 2007; Sabri, Merkel, Tichomirowa 2016.

257 Wilson 2002, 24–9.

4.7 *Post-Roman Water Culture*

In Late Antiquity, water culture naturally continued throughout the lands of the former Roman Empire, but perhaps not built in the same degree or intensity as before. For example, in North Africa, the existing water technologies and infrastructure lasted through the Vandal invasions and the Byzantine period; however, new aqueduct systems were extremely rare.[258] In the city of Rome, during the Gothic siege of 537–538, all the aqueducts were cut, in order to force the city to surrender.[259] After the siege, only four of the 11 aqueducts were repaired, and it was not until the Baroque period that the popes were able to begin restoring some of the aqueducts in earnest.[260]

Recently, more research has been conducted on Late Antique water systems. The aqueducts of the site of Gortyn (Crete) have been published by Elisabetta Giorgi.[261] In addition to documenting the aqueducts of the Imperial period, Giorgi has extensively explored the final phase of the aqueduct there, which is dated to the sixth and seventh centuries. As Gortyn was the prominent provincial capital of Crete and Cyrenaica in the Imperial period, her work has shown how the city changed in the Late Antique period. By the sixth and seventh centuries, the monumental city center, which was once full of civic and religious structures, was turned into an industrial zone that needed more water.[262] Thus, aqueduct studies can demonstrate ways in which urban centers evolve, as water systems were adapted to shifts in the use of space. Furthermore, Jordan Pickett has studied water infrastructure systems of the eastern Mediterranean (300–800 CE), in a similar manner to Giorgi.[263]

Further, modern scholarship has increasingly focused on fountains of the Late Antique period. Ine Jacobs and Richard have surveyed the Late Antique fountains of Asia Minor.[264] They have been able to demonstrate in this period that, while already existing fountains were maintained where possible, new structures were also constructed, albeit more modest and cost-effective

258 Wilson 2012, 5.

259 For more on the geological aspects of the waters of Rome from antiquity until the present day, see Pandolfi (2008).

260 Wilson 2008, 298. For more on the water of the city of Rome in the Baroque period, see the monograph of Rinne (2010), which not only gives a social history of the aqueducts, fountains, and Tiber River in that period, but also highlights the importance of the engineering aspects of the water infrastructure of the city—thus drastically transforming modern Rome.

261 Giorgi 2016.

262 Giorgi 2007, 314.

263 Pickett 2015.

264 Jacobs and Richard 2012.

than their predecessors, prioritizing the need to conserve water in an uncertain period, when unknown political or social changes could impact the distribution of water. Other scholars are continuing to reexamine previously studied fountains throughout the eastern Mediterranean, from Gortyn to Constantinople, demonstrating that fountains were still an important part of life in the Late Antique period.[265]

The water of Constantinople has also recently received a great deal of attention in scholarship. Constantinople as a city lacks a natural source of potable drinking water.[266] With its position as the 'New Rome,' it is believed that Constantinople copied elements of the water system of Rome, although probably not of the same sophistication.[267] Constantinople was first supplied with water under Hadrian, and later its main aqueduct was completed by the emperor Valens in 373 CE, bringing water from Thrace, at a length of nearly 268 km.[268] Over the next few centuries, the aqueduct continued to grow in length to accommodate the fifth-century growth of the city—making it one of the longest aqueducts in the ancient world, reaching nearly 971 m long.[269] This aqueduct remained in continuous use until at least the time of Justinian, with later disruptions in the seventh century (due to neglect), and a restoration by Constantine V in 767 that provided water until at least the First Crusade (1095–1099).[270] Water supplied a number of structures throughout the capital, including baths, monumental fountains, etc., many of which are mentioned in the fifth-century *Notitia urbis Constantinopolitanae*.[271] Water was also stored in a network of 150 cisterns throughout the city, constructed with freestanding columns (and not the pier system used in Rome); the surplus of water stored in Constantinople provided an element of security in increasingly volatile times.[272]

265 For example, see Stephenson and Hedlund (2016) and Longfellow (2016) on the monumental fountains of Constantinople, and Longfellow (2018) on the second phase of the nymphaeum of the so-called Praetorium of Gortyn. See also Sodini, Kozelj, and Wurch-Koželj (2016) on the nymphaeum in a Late Antique house on the island of Thasos.

266 Crow 2012a, 53.

267 Ward-Perkins 2012, 65. See also Grig and Kelly (2012) for an overview on examining the cities of Rome and Constantinople together.

268 Crow 2012a, 37–38. The aqueduct system of Constantinople was extensively surveyed, mapped, and studied by Crow, Bardill, and Bayliss (2008), bringing to light unknown elements of the system itself.

269 Crow 2012a, 37.

270 Crow 2012b, 135.

271 See Matthews (2012) on the *Notitia urbis Constantinopolitanae*.

272 Crow 2012a, 41.

Over the course of the fifth and sixth centuries, water administration and legislation became more codified. The Theodosian and Justinianic Law Codes provided for: "(1) maintenance of the system outside of the city and regulation of water for agricultural uses; (2) distribution and allocation within the city; (3) maintaining and financing the system."[273] Of primary importance for the whole system was that it had provisions for public water. Over the course of the Late Antique period and into the Byzantine period, there were a number of offices tied to water maintenance, including the *hydrophylacae*, the *logothetes ton hydaton*, and the ninth century *komites hydaton*, the 'counts of the waters,' a branch of the state's revenue and tax office.[274] Despite the similarities with Rome, some scholars still debate whether the Constantinople system was actually modeled after the one in Rome. For example, only one lead *fistula* has been discovered in Constantinople, unlike the hundreds of Rome.[275] Regardless, the water infrastructure system of Constantinople was tied to the emperor and his court, as "water was a key resource for displaying power, expressed through the provision of free-flowing fountains for the population of the city and for urban baths and *nymphaea*: traditional components of classical euergetism."[276]

The Romans laid the foundations for the use and enjoyment of water through the Late Antique and Byzantine periods. It has been noted that in these later periods, engineers relied on earlier Roman technological advances, thus there was no great need for further innovations in aqueduct or bath technologies, for example.[277] Still, water played an important role in the Byzantine period, especially as the city of Constantinople flourished, while other urban centers of the West began to fail. A recent conference (the proceedings of which were published in the collected volume, *Fountains and Water Culture in Byzantium*) discussed, among other things: the role of water in the Byzantine Empire; the use of water and sound in fountains; the decline of *thermae* by the ninth century (as many were converted into churches); and the use of water in Christian doctrine and theology, such as the cult of the Virgin Mary as the *Zoodochos Pege*, the 'Life-Giving Source.'[278] Scholars are also revisiting previously accepted

273 Crow 2012a, 42.

274 Crow 2012a, 36, 43, 50.

275 This of course may be ascribed to the regional trend of using terracotta conduits in the region. For more on the *fistula*, see De Kleijn (2016, 55, 58–59). For more on the find spot of this one *fistula*, which was part of the fountain of the famous Serpent Column, see Stephenson (2016, 109–11).

276 Crow 2012b, 134.

277 Lewis 2007, 375.

278 On the sound of fountains, see Dauterman Maguire (2016); on baths, see Magdalino (2016, 142) and Kullberg (2016); on the *Zoodochos Pege*, see Bodin (2016) and Kimmelfield (2016).

notions, such as the connection of baths with baptism. While Roman bathing culture was habitual and daily, baptism was a singular and spiritually transformative experience.[279] This research demonstrates the multivalent nature of water in cultures after the Romans, showing its importance beyond the need for mere survival. In a new Christian context, water took on a more eternally nourishing, spiritual aspect.

5 Empire-Wide Trends and Phenomena

There are a number of features that are considered to be characteristic of the ancient Roman city. By the time of the High Empire, it is clear that there was a set of 'requirements' that one expected from a city to provide comfort, order, and security. In an often quoted passage, Pausanias, describing Panopeus of Phocia (Greece), is shocked that the site has the status of a *polis*, as the inhabitants have "no government offices, no gymnasium, no theater, no market-place, no water descending to a fountain, but live in bare shelters just like mountain cabins, right on a ravine."[280] Similarly, in his oration on Rome, Aelius Aristides described the cities of the provinces as "full of gymnasia, fountains, gateways, temples, handicrafts, and schools."[281]

The passages of Pausanias and Aristides both cite water-displays within a litany of necessary structures for a Roman city.[282] This raises questions about empire-wide trends in water consumption. Currently, there is no complete modern discussion of such trends. Thus, one must piece together patterns of water usage from disparate studies across the empire in order to begin to understand differences that can be discerned from the available evidence. The most salient differences can be attributed to climatic conditions and indigenous social practices. Regardless, even if modes or rates of consumption varied across the different climatic and geographic regions of the empire, Roman water culture was ubiquitous and far-reaching.

---

279 Kullberg 2016, 155–57.

280 Paus. 10.4.1. (Trans. W.H.S. Jones). γε οὐκ ἀρχεῖα οὐ γυμνάσιόν ἐστιν, οὐ θέατρον οὐκ ἀγορὰν ἔχουσιν, οὐχ ὕδωρ κατερχόμενον ἐς κρήνην, ἀλλὰ ἐν στέγαις κοίλαις κατὰ τὰς καλύβας μάλιστα τὰς ἐν τοῖς ὄρεσιν, ἐνταῦθα οἰκοῦσιν ἐπὶ χαράδρᾳ. See Alcock (1995) and Rubinstein (1995) for a discussion of the nature of the *polis* by the time of Pausanias, with special emphasis on this passage.

281 Aristid. *Or.* 26.97 (Trans. Behr 1981). πάντα δὲ μεστά γυμνασίων, κρήνων, προπυλαίων, νεῶν, δημιουργιῶν, διδασκάλων. See also Thomas (2007, 121) and Pont (2010, 170).

282 Aristides is known to have written in other instances on water, such as in the extant fragments of a panegyric he gave on the waters of Pergamon (Jones 1991).

Most of modern Europe is part of the former empire, which has a temperate climate, with healthy rainfalls. There are, however, many other drier climates in the empire, including those characterized as hyper-arid, arid, and semi-arid. 'Hyper-arid' regions are those associated with the deserts of Africa and the Middle East.[283] 'Semi-arid' denotes climatic conditions in which occasional, severe droughts jeopardize the successful cultivation of crops and livestock, such as in parts of the Iberian Peninsula, Turkey, and North Africa. The Roman Empire also included regions with true 'arid' climates, characterized by a desert-like, harsh and regular lack of rainfall, such as the modern countries located on the so-called 'Arid Belt,' including Libya, Egypt, Sudan, Jordan, Yemen, Oman, United Arab Emirates, Iran, Turkmenistan, etc.[284]

Roman water infrastructure was present in practically the whole of the empire but was used in various ways depending on the needs prescribed by these drastically different climates. For example, the semi-arid areas of North Africa, hosted an extensive network of aqueducts and cisterns, as Wilson has documented.[285] Wilson's work demonstrates how inhabitants of this region ensured sufficient water supplies throughout all seasons: systems for regulating reservoir usage (especially for heavy water users such as baths), as well as taps and stopcocks at points of use (not simply at reservoirs), which allowed for greater control of the water. Further, Richard's study of fountains in the Roman East has shown that, while the fountains were monumental in scale, they operated on relatively small amounts of water.[286] In a similar vein, Christoph Ohlig has outlined the differences in domestic water usage practices between Pompeii and Colonia Ulpia Traiana (Xanten, Germany), two sites that have very different climatic conditions.[287]

Societal practices are also of great importance in considering differences in water consumption across the empire. Zena Kamash has demonstrated that

---

283 For more on drylands and the archaeology that can be undertook there, see the collected volume of Barker and Gilbertson (2000).

284 For more on the 'Arid Belt,' especially in the context of the ancient world, see the collected volume of Liverani (2003), which explores life at arid sites in the Roman Empire. The volume was the product of a conference hosted by the Centro Interuniversario di Ricerca sulla civiltà e l'ambiente del Sahara antico (CIRSA) of the Università di Roma 'La Sapienza.' The group strives to study life diachronically in arid lands. See also various contributions in Franconi's 2017 volume on fluvial landscapes, which investigate climate change's impact on ancient river landscapes.

285 Wilson 2001.

286 Richard 2012, 173–76; see also Richard (2016a). See Rogers (2015, 413–14) for more on the regional trends in water-displays across the empire.

287 Ohlig 2012.

although water-related technologies were successfully implemented across the Roman Near East, some were not as popular as others.[288] Among the most successful were stepped-dams, bridges, and bathing complexes, while lead pipes, water-displays, and latrines apparently had only limited appeal.[289] As lead pipes were not universally adopted across the region, cisterns were popular in domestic contexts, which explains the limited popularity of water-displays in the home.[290] Another reason is that homes in the East were not meant to be as publicly accessible as their counterparts in the West, which often featured views through the atrium to beautiful water-displays.[291] Bathing complexes achieved noticeable success in the third century CE, while latrines achieved a limited popularity only in the fourth century. Kamash attributes the success of baths to the daily necessity of bathing (and the social interactions that happened at the baths), while latrines might have only received limited success due to local religious concerns against the exposure of the nude human body.[292] Surely there are other such regional socially-constructed distinctions in water use to discover still.

Much remains to be done in terms of regional trends of water usage across the Roman Empire, but a foundation has been laid in the modern scholarship. In order to ensure stable and reliable water sources, local populations readily adopted Roman water infrastructure systems, which could be implemented to varying degrees based on local needs. Again, water culture is not monolithic, and it can easily adapt to local concerns, while still allowing local populations to enjoy the myriad of benefits water provides.

6 Water Culture and Its Implications

The previous discussion of the various aspects of water usage by the Romans has touched on many aspects of Roman society at large. It will be helpful, then, to examine the employment and manipulation of water by the Romans more holistically, outlining trends in how water impacted the wider conceptions of Roman culture. Given the ubiquity of water in the Roman world, many aspects of water culture in Roman society overlap. This fact, however, helps to

288 Kamash 2010; 2012.

289 Kamash 2012, 83, 90–1.

290 The site of Dura-Europos has no evidence of private water-displays, which Kamash attributes to the use of cisterns (2012, 86–7).

291 Kamash 2012, 87. On western examples and their sight lines, see Rogers (2013, 158).

292 Kamash 2012, 88–9.

illustrate the importance and dominance water had on how an ancient Roman lived, regardless of where he or she resided in the empire.

6.1 *Power*

There is a natural power behind being able to harness water and use it for other purposes. Previous studies of the political and social power of water have been general, and they have not sufficiently expressed the complexities of the different aspects of the Romans' use of water.[293] In the Greek world various tyrants, who were known for completing water-related projects to curry favor with their people, were able to create 'spaces of power,' translating political power into the surrounding artificial built environment.[294] These types of spaces continued into the Roman Empire, when symbolic forms of architecture (e.g., the arch, specific types of public buildings) signified the domination of the Romans.[295] Indeed, by employing expected architectural forms, a benefactor or a community could show their ties to Rome, despite their diverse backgrounds and social statuses.[296]

There is an innate power that one witnesses in flowing water, no matter the context. A trip to the Baroque-era Trevi Fountain in Rome, with its resplendent decorative program and impressive water flow, never ceases to amaze even the modern veteran visitor of the city. The same feeling can certainly be expected to have been felt by ancient Romans, especially those in semi-arid climates, where the display of water would be a stark juxtaposition with the surrounding dry landscape.[297] The water-related structures of the Romans can be considered symbols of conspicuous consumption, visual statements and reminders to all of the ability and resources of the Romans. Indeed, as it will be seen in the ensuing discussion, flowing water in fountains and baths, and its associated built structures (e.g., aqueducts), can invoke the power of the Romans. More monumental architectural forms of water, as opposed to more utilitarian forms (e.g., watermills), demonstrate the political and social power of their builders. In this context, this section explores imperial and private benefactions of water, private and civic status, Roman dominance over nature, and rhetoric.

Benefactions of water were omnipresent throughout the Roman world. The emperor himself could dedicate aqueducts, fountains, and bath complexes,

293 Tölle-Kastenbein 1990, 177–86; Malissard 1994, 246–308.

294 Arvanitis 2008, 1.

295 Thomas 2007, 150.

296 Thomas 2007, 7.

297 Piras 2006.

in his name and for the people. These types of structures visually signaled to users political power, and thus a political ideology, behind their construction. Unlike drains underneath the streets, for example, aqueducts, fountains, and bath complexes were tangible. Further, structures like these could be enjoyed on a personal level within an urban environment. And, naturally, the same structures were also funded by private individuals wishing to emulate the emperor and support their local communities.[298] Benefactions could easily elevate the status of a place, as was the case with Athens and other cities in Greece, where Hadrian dedicated a number of aqueducts and fountains during his reign. Athens, especially as it was not in the same high position it held in the Classical period, benefitted immensely from this benefaction, owing to the emperor's philhellene tendencies.[299] Indeed, the political and cultural benefits that these structures provided to those living in Greece often outweighed the blatant elements of conspicuous consumption of the structures. There have also been questions of how patronage was directed. Did a particular class of water-related building projects originate in Rome and go to the provinces, or vice versa?[300] Regardless, there was a concerted effort to offer public benefactions throughout the Roman world, often on different scales, that made water publicly available to all.

Status connected with water-related architecture has been much discussed in modern scholarship. Especially in areas where water was physically scarce, such as North Africa and Asia Minor, civic water projects could immediately lend status to a community.[301] These settlements were tapping into a wider Roman desire to have access to water, which the Roman imperial framework allowed and supported. Aqueducts, for example, could provide an element of civic pride for urban settlements.[302] The status afforded these cities led, in turn, to competition among cities for bigger and better forms of water-related structures.[303] For example, the Nymphaeum of the Tritons at Hierapolis and

298 The benefactions of public fountains by the emperor and members of the local élite are explored most fully by Longfellow (2011).

299 Leigh 1998; Koloski-Ostrow 2001, 7; Longfellow 2011, 107–39.

300 For example, Longfellow (2011, 164–82) argues that the form of the monumental Septizodium fountain of Rome can be derived from the provinces, especially given that Septimius Severus, its benefactor, was from Africa.

301 Wilson 1995; Piras 2000.

302 Koloski-Ostrow 2001, 4.

303 Dorl-Klingenschmid 2006; Thomas 2007, 127. For more on competition between cities in Asia Minor, see: Robert 1977; Heller 2006; Kuhn 2013. See also the recent article of Lendon (2015), who argues that the influx of large-scale fountains in Asia Minor could be attributed to the élite education of local young men, as the monumental fountain type and its

the nymphaeum of Laodicaea-on-the-Lycus, both of Severan date, were built in competition with each other, particularly as they are both of monumental in scale (well over 40 m long each).[304]

Status was also evidently elevated for those who had water in their private dwellings. Throughout the Roman Empire, the ability to obtain a private water right meant that an owner had to petition the emperor in Rome or the local civic authorities.[305] Thus, private water concessions would then allow an owner to use and display water, automatically elevating his or her status.[306] Some examples, such as in the House of the Vestals in Pompeii, demonstrate how owners, once they had access to water, could complete renovations to their homes that could incorporate new ways of displaying water, keeping up with the fashions of time.[307] While most water in the Roman house could be used for utilitarian and practical purposes, there is some evidence that not all of the water was saved for secondary use, again, demonstrating the status of the owner, who could have a surplus of water.[308] In relation to status, flowing water inside a domestic space also illustrated the wealth of the owner.[309] Edmund Thomas, in a recent reanalysis of the Augustan-era Villa Claudia at Anguillara Sabazia (northwest of Rome), has shown that the impressive water-displays there mimic the architecture of Augustus' Naumachia in Rome, illustrating the wealth of the villa's owner and the resources that he or she was able to muster to construct the water-displays there.[310] Thus, particularly in the visible display of water in domestic spaces, owners were able to declare their elevated status to all.

Both the benefaction of, and the status afforded to, individuals and communities by water-related projects share an underlying theme: dominance over nature. Given the destructive nature of water, Romans were able to construct structures and enact safeguards against water's forces, such as river flooding.[311] Nicholas Purcell has demonstrated in a series of articles the strong nature of

connection to the water supply offered a new ways to teach the art of rhetoric in the High Imperial period.

304 Longfellow 2011, 189–90; Rogers 2015, 252, 259–60.

305 Bruun 2012c. See also above, 18.

306 Schmölder-Veit 2009, 161. See Rogers (2013, 158) on the lines of sight from the streets of Pompeii into the interiors of homes, so that passers-by could see water-displays therein.

307 Jones and Robinson 2005.

308 Zarmakoupi 2014, 146.

309 Compare with Koloski-Ostrow 2001.

310 Thomas 2012.

311 See above, 10–11, especially with Bruun 1992.

the Romans' relationship with water—an element that comes from elsewhere, flows elsewhere, and with which an individual's experience is usually fleeting.[312] The concerted effort of Romans to control water, especially over the course of the empire, became an integral part of the administrative apparatus of the empire, improving its survival.[313] Purcell states that water "had a vital contribution to make: directly through the basic problem of conceptualizing a mobile element in a wide environment, and indirectly through the complex cultural and legal associations connected with each watery landscape."[314] Romans then, in their 'rhetoric of control,' to borrow a phrase of Purcell, were successfully able to demonstrate their power over nature, while still supplying a vital and pleasurable element necessary for their subjects.[315]

Perhaps one of the greatest benefits of the Romans' relationship with water was making it publicly available, while still maintaining a certain air of exclusivity. While even the Greeks had legal regulations that provided for the public water supply, the Romans continued this tradition, but on a much grander scale—and at a time when private water rights were legally controlled, imbuing such imperial projects with all the more prestige value. Even the 11 aqueducts of the city of Rome can illustrate this point, given the sheer population of the city, which would require vast amounts of water. While there was public access to water throughout the empire, often at local public fountains or in the public baths, there was still an exclusivity of water usage, usually by the emperor and those who had private water rights. Longfellow, discussing water-displays, says that "aquatic displays, ranging from the small jets ringing Pompeian impluvia to the Augustan Meta Sudans in the heart of Rome, celebrated water in a manner that symbolized the bounty of the empire, as well as the political power, social status, and wealth that were wished for by many but possessed by few."[316] Thus, the divide between those who had access to different types of water use, whether publicly or privately, helped to delineate levels notions of power in the Roman Empire—thereby reinforcing the hierarchies that structured the empire's social organization.

---

312 Purcell 1996, 200. See Purcell (1996 and 2012). In a similar vein, see Kleiner (1991) on the Roman triumph over nature, particularly water, through bridge-building.

313 Purcell 1996, 193, 207.

314 Purcell 1996, 203–204.

315 See Purcell 1996, 206.

316 Longfellow 2011, 28.

6.2 *Aesthetics*

> Haec utilitas haec amoenitas deficitur aqua salienti, sed puteos ac potius fontes habet; sunt enim in summo.
>
> PLINY, *EP.* 2.17.25

> Only one thing is needed to complete the amenities and beauty of the house—running water; but there are wells, or rather springs, for they are very near the surface.
>
> TRANS. B. RADICE

The aesthetics of water are infinite. Pliny the Younger in his *Letter* about his Laurentine Villa expresses the idea that a house is made better through the use of *running* water, not just water that can be found in a well. He goes on in the *Letter* to describe the space's numerous decorative water features, which clearly gave him and his guests delight and pleasure. The luxury and sensual nature of the flowing water evidently enhanced the various spaces throughout the villa, vitalizing them. While a Roman villa certainly did not need to have water-displays and running water, these features were certainly desirable, making the complex even more enjoyable.

While water can be aesthetically pleasing on its own in nature, when it is controlled and subjected to architectural forms, it can take on new meanings. For example, when an ancient Roman saw an aqueduct arcade, he or she could think first of the running water inside (*utilitas*), while still admiring its external beauty of superimposed arcades (*amoenitas*). Moreover, given that many aqueducts terminated in urban water-displays, an aqueduct out in the country could also be viewed metonymically: an extraurban signifier of the powerful public building projects taking place in the city.[317] Further, the forms of architecture that water-related structures in the Roman world adopted would take on empire-wide symbolic meanings of a shared identity.[318] Thus, aqueducts employed iconic arcaded forms, which, of course, while aesthetically pleasing, were also highly functional. Bath complexes by the start of the empire took on canonical architectural forms that allowed bathers to progress through the various cold to hot rooms. The imperial baths of the city of Rome, with their sheer size, not only spoke of the monumental architectural forms, but also the power behind the imperial commission. Fountains came in different sizes

317 Wilson 1998, 93.

318 Thomas 2007, 127.

and shapes, but the large-scale façade fountains found throughout the empire demonstrate a shared architectural vocabulary that, with the addition of flowing water and decoration, created splashy spaces of luxury.

Part of the aesthetic experience behind many water-related structures, such as fountains and baths, were their decorative programs. Precious materials, such as imported marbles in the imperial baths of Rome, illustrated the stretches of the empire—and the ability that the Romans had to obtain these exotic materials. Sculptural decoration of both baths and fountains illustrated programs that stressed subjects related to abundance, mythology, history, and patronage/imperial ideology. For example, the Baths of Caracalla in Rome, resplendent in imported marble on its floors and walls, was full of sculpture. Images of Hercules not only invoked a mythical figure, especially as a protector of hot springs, but also Caracalla's own connections to Hercules.[319] Thus, the decoration of structures associated with water could add to the aesthetic beauty of the complex itself, while also hinting at other connections to water, myth, and history.

In the same vein, the symbolism behind water and its use in water-related structures is multivalent. First and foremost, water symbolizes purity.[320] Water's ability to cleanse is crucial for its role in Greco-Roman religion, in particular, as an ancient had to wash his or her hands upon entering a religious space.[321] Mythology is also full of water-related subjects. For example, river gods and nymphs can serve as symbols for water, especially in a decorative program of a fountain or private house. Depictions of the Tiber River, which could be found throughout the empire, were symbols for not only water, but also a wider sense of identity tied to the capital.[322] As was discussed in the previous section, water, especially in private spaces, invokes luxury and status.[323] As villas have been described as places of self-promotion and social difference, the addition of running water can only have elevated the status of a villa, especially in combination with other decorative programs.[324]

319 DeLaine 1997, 78–80; Piranomonte 2012, 72. On a related note, see Salowey (1994) on the role and meaning of Hercules on Roman waterworks of the Peloponnese.

320 Tölle-Kastenbein 1990, 14; Topták 2009; Aristodemou 2011, 192–96.

321 *ThesCRA* 2.3a.IV.A (s.v., Purificazione, Romana, Mezzi impiegati nelle purificazioni, liquidi e uguenti; V. Saladino).

322 Meyers 2009; Tayor 2009.

323 Zarmakoupi 2014, 141, 147.

324 On this conception of the Roman villa, see Zarmakoupi (2014, 213).

6.3 *Water as Spectacle*

Roman entertainments, especially in the empire, included aquatic spectacles. Among the various water-related spectacles in the Roman world were: *naumachiae* (mock sea battles); aquatic *venationes*; and hydromimes (shows in pools that included choreographed swimming).[325] These spectacles were different than the other shows put on in the arenas of the Roman world. And because of that fact, either new structures had to be constructed (e.g., *naumachiae*) or pre-existing buildings had to be altered to accommodate large amounts of water. For example, in the latter part of the empire, theater orchestras were walled up and waterproofed to allow for pools, the *kolymbethra*.[326] A number of these aquatic spectacles appear to illustrate historical battles, especially of the distant past, such as the battle between Corcyra and Corinth of 434 BCE, which Dio reports was staged in 80 CE in the Flavian Amphitheater of Rome.[327] Kathleen Coleman demonstrates that these aquatic spectacles were lavish, which added to the perceived authenticity of the events by spectators.[328] Further, the Romans did not restrict themselves to mock naval battles, but transformed Roman pantomime into hydromimes, or tableaus set in marine contexts.[329] Water, in a sense, helped to create indelible experiences for Romans throughout the empire. Thus, the concept and performance of aquatic 'spectacle' can inform new discussions about the nature of the Roman tastes.

The Roman spectacle has received a great deal of scholarly attention in the last decade or so. The English word derives from the Latin *spectaculum*, which, for the Romans had a variety of meanings, including a sight or manifestation, entertainment in the form of a performance, or the structures associated with entertainment.[330] The last definition is the most interesting for the present discussion. In Classical Latin, when *spectaculum* is used in the plural, *spectacula*, it is understood to mean "the places occupied by spectators in a theater, etc."[331] From at least the censorship of C. Maenius (318 BCE) until the

325 The most exhaustive resource on these aquatic spectacles of the Romans is Berlan-Bajard (2006), along with Coleman (1993). For more on *naumachiae*, see Cariou (2009). See also Traversari (1960) for a discussion of aquatic spectacles of Late Antiquity, with reconstruction drawings of entertainment complexes complete with hydromimes (by Italo Gismondi).

326 On the *kolymbethra*, see especially Berlan-Bajard (2006, 255–78).

327 Dio 67.25.3. See Coleman's discussion of this spectacle (1993, especially 60–2).

328 Coleman 1993, 73.

329 Coleman 1993, 49.

330 D'Arms 1999, 301.

331 *OLD*² s.v., Spectaculum, 3. The associated literature for this definition is as follows: Pl. *Cur.* 647; Cic. *Har.* 22, *Sest.* 124; Vitr. 5.6.2; Liv. 1.35.9, 45.1.2; Ov. *Met.* 10.668; Calp. *Ecl.* 7.23; Tac. *Ann.* 14.13; Juv. 8.205; Fest. p. 84M; Suet. *Cal.* 31.

time of Pompey, it is known that in the Forum Romanum, there were *spectacula* made of wood.[332] The dedicatory inscription of the amphitheater of Pompeii, dated to about 70 BCE, describes the structure as a *spectacula*, not an amphitheater (*CIL* 10.852). This naturally raises the question of whether the *spectacula* were in fact the buildings themselves, or the entertainments taking place in those spaces.[333] Such early use of *spectacula* is important here. Entertainment-related spaces could in fact be public spaces at large, an idea which at first glance might be jarring to a modern audience that is used to entertainments taking place in specially constructed spaces. Spectacle, then, in the Roman world can encompass a variety of different places and cannot be limited to just one type of space.

Spectacle can be defined in a number of ways. Cultural performances, as defined by sociologist John MacAloon, include spectacles, rituals, and festivals.[334] Diane Favro, building upon this idea, argues that "spectacles are expansive, open-ended events that evoke an array of emotions."[335] In a similar manner, spectacles should amaze "by virtue of [their] nature, scale, or novelty."[336] It follows easily that spectacles are often first associated with entertainment, such as the famous *munera* of the Romans.[337] The *munera* provided performative events for the Roman public, and the populace would deem imperial *munera* successful based on their lavishness—for example, by the incorporation of exotic animals in the arena. The use of flowing water could potentially then be considered an entertainment, intended to delight the public with its ability to control and display water in innovative ways.

---

332 Welch 2007, 32–3, 43–58. Welch describes the development of the *spectacula* in the Forum Romanum over the course of the middle to the end of the Republic (43–58).

333 Indeed, *spectacula* is used until Vitruvius first uses the neologism, *amphitheatrum* (Rawson 1987, 86–7). Davies (1997, 121, no. 83) argues that *spectacula* here would have only alluded to the entertainments taking place in the amphitheater, not the physical space, namely because of the attestation of *amphitheatrum* was by Vitruvius (1.7.1).

334 MacAloon 1966.

335 Favro 1999, 205. See also Wiles (2003) for more on the performativity of space, including sacred, processional, and public spaces, among others. His discussion is tied intimately to conceptions of performativity and theatrical space throughout history.

336 Edmondson 1999, 77. Edmondson explores the relationship with literary works and spectacles, especially how they both tend to follow certain patterns to be intelligible to viewers.

337 See the work of Beacham (1991 and 1999) for more on the development of spectacle and entertainment in the empire, including how the emperor asserted his dominance through entertainments and how public life becomes more of a theatrical performance in the empire.

Entertainments in the Roman world were sponsored by one party, the benefactor, and viewed by other parties, the audience. The benefactors, given their economic ability to fund a spectacle, asserted their power and prestige through this benefaction, often gaining support, whether political or otherwise, from those in the audience, many of whom might be their own clients.[338] In a sense, entertainments were a way in which Romans of the élite classes could define their relationship with their subordinates, using these spectacles as "vehicles of self-representation," by showing their audience the way they wished to be viewed.[339] Often, the entertainments put on during the empire would have pushed the boundaries of known and accepted spectacle, as Coleman demonstrates in her discussion of the aquatic displays of the Early Empire (e.g., the *naumachiae*, or ship battles, of Augustus).[340] Such displays used entertainment in novel ways that would have been enjoyable to its audience, causing them to remember the event and the benefactor.

An important Roman office connected with spectacle is that of aedile. Because the duties of the aediles originally included those of the *cura urbis* (office of the city, connected with the urban prefect), *cura annonae* (office of grain allotments), and *cura ludorum sollemnium* (office of the games and religious ceremonies), this meant that the aediles supervised public building, such as the upkeep of temples and water supply, and put on spectacles for the populace. In the city of Rome, the aedileship was mainly relevant in the time before Augustus' internal government reorganization, including the institution of the *cura aquarum*, which managed water; in Italian and provincial cities, however, the aedile's functions did not diminish.[341] It is the fact that aediles were intimately tied to public works and spectacle is interesting here because both often featured impressive water-related projects. Agrippa in 33 BCE, when he was installing the Aqua Virgo and the accompanying *castella, lacus*, and *salientes*, held the office of aedile. In addition, extant inscriptions occasionally reveal that aediles sponsored the building or restoration of water-displays. For example, two aediles, perhaps in the Early Empire, in Urbinum Mataurense (modern Urbino, Italy), restored a *saliens* there after four years of disrepair (*CIL* 8.2631). One can imagine that the *saliens* provided not only necessary drinking water for the people of Urbinum, but also a display of flowing

338 D'Arms 1999, 308–309. Bell (2004) believes that Greek and Roman public figures used spectacle in their own self-presentation to their audiences. Coleman (2006) offers a pointed critique of Bell's articulation and presentation of his argument.

339 Beacham 1991, x; Kondoleon 1999, 321.

340 Coleman 1993, 69.

341 For an overview of the aediles in the Republic, see Drogula (2000).

water in the street, which—especially after a four year hiatus—would have noticeably revitalized the street itself. The connection between the office of the aedile and water projects is, in the very least, suggestive of the nature of Roman public water works, and thus a link can also be drawn between the entertainment-related ventures of the aedile and his support of water features that had the potential to act as spectacles.

It is also important to consider the ephemerality of spectacle. Spectacles are part of cultural performance, which includes rituals and festivals, all of which often occur over the course of a day or series of days, relegating them to the memories of the audience following completion. While the audience certainly enjoyed and craved these public spectacles and entertainments, after they were done there was no physical reminder of them, with the exception of structures specifically built to house them or souvenirs purchased at the event.[342] The water flowing through a fountain, for example, is ephemeral. But because the structure is permanent, the ephemeral nature of flowing water is superceded by the fountain. Despite the fact that the water drains away, the memory of the flowing water in a permanent structure continues on in the minds of viewers. In a sense, given the lasting nature of the permanent water-display, investment in that spectacle will last much longer for the patron, longer than the single day the traditional spectacle took. Water-displays then effectively combine ephemerality and permanency to create a unique style of spectacle in the Roman world.

Finally, spectacle is intimately tied to the space that it occupies. The place in which spectacle occurs would surely evoke for its audience different associations:

> including historic activities that have occurred in the same place; the way it may have been specially fashioned or altered to take on unaccustomed symbolic meaning; and its location relative to other areas of urban space and their significance.[343]

Favro expands this idea by asserting that "ancient urban locales played a part in the creation, presentation, and interpretation of public performances" and that "Roman urban sites augmented self-awareness likewise by serving as

342 For more on souvenirs in the Roman period, especially for tourists, see essays in the edited volume of Schmitz and Sieler (2013). An ephemeral spectacle, such as a triumph, could be captured in durable forms, such as on the Gemma Augustea. For more, see Kuttner (1999, 97 and 118).

343 Bartsch 1994, 24.

repositories of human memory."[344] The locations where spectacles took place, then, would not only have been vital in the creation of the actual entertainment, but also would have created a long-lasting memory for the audience, associated with that particular location. For example, one can imagine approaching the Severan Septizodium in Rome, with its imposing three-storied façade, sumptuous statuary program, and cascading water. Coming from the south, one would enter the city at the Porta Capena, with the monumental backdrop of the fountain, adjacent to the Circus Maximus and the Palatine Hill. Passers-by, not only thirsty for the water, also made memories of approaching the fountain when they entered the city—illustrating the wealth and grandeur of the imperial capital.

Further, the Roman street offers another example of spectacle. Barbara Kellum asserts that the "the street was the pivotal performative arena in a visual culture where viewership was active and confrontational."[345] Here, however, the line between the spectacle and the spectator begins to break down, as the spectator becomes an active participant in the spectacle of the street. Unlike the entertainments that might occur in the arena, the street, with its walls covered with paintings and graffiti, would have been a spectacle in and of itself, and a place intimately familiar to the inhabitants of that space. Thus, place is integral to the spectacle, not only providing the space for the performance to occur, but also creating associated memories and new performance spaces for its audiences.

The use of water has not been included in the modern scholarship on spectacle, and yet, as has been demonstrated here, there are numerous reasons to draw this connection.[346] There is an audience for water-related structures, especially fountains—those who enjoy the aesthetic and utilitarian aspects of the structure. With the audience, then, naturally comes the benefactor, who paid for the structure, helping to define the relationships between those with power and money and those dependent on them. Unlike other Roman spectacles, a fountain, for example, is not ephemeral, just as the amphitheater in Pompeii, known as a *spectacula* in an inscription, is not ephemeral, either. Water-displays are more than just a *monumentum*, a built structure that can

344 Favro 1999, 205.

345 Kellum 1999, 283.

346 Malissard (1994, 88–102) does use the term 'spectacle' to describe *naumachiae*, clepysdras (water clocks), hydraulic organs, and decorative fountains, but fails to offer a theoretical discussion of the term. For a discussion of theatricality and spectacle associated with Roman water, see Rogers (2015, 359–68).

aid in the preservation of memories.[347] It might be suggested, then, that the water-display, like other permanent physical structures devoted to entertainment, could certainly be considered a *spectaculum*, too. Indeed, as mentioned previously, many fountains, especially those grand façades found in the Roman East, suggest architectural forms also found in theaters.[348] Further, the fountain is tied to place, given that it is a 'living' part of the urban landscape, especially in that water constantly flows through it, making it a dynamic structure of the city. As memory is tied to place, the audience would have created memories of the water-display by interacting with the structure over time. Indeed, in the Roman city, because the fountain is located in the streets, an inherently performative place, the lines between the audience and the spectacle are blurred, allowing for the audience to become active participants in the spectacle that is the water-display, whether enjoying the fountain itself or collecting water from its basins. While not a traditional Roman spectacle, such as the *ludi gladiatori* in the arena, the actual water-display of the fountain would have nevertheless created a spectacle. And by extension, other water-related structures, such as aqueducts and baths, can be incorporated into a discussion of spectacle.

6.4 *Shared Cultural Experience of Water*

Charles Moore, the modern architect who designed a number of water-related installations in his career, captured the essence of water that transcends time and different societies: "[The] *architecture of water* [can be defined as] what physical laws govern its behavior, how the liquid acts and reacts with our senses, and, most of all, how its symbolism relates to us as human beings."[349] Indeed, such an assertion can also be associated with Romans and their interactions with water. Further, this experience translates easily into shared experiences that the Romans had with water, regardless of their time or location within the empire. The aim of this section is not to generalize about a large swath of geography over centuries with countless inhabitants, but to highlight salient points regarding the shared Roman cultural experience of water that

347 Feldherr (1998, especially 21–5, 31–5) explores how Livy's *History* is like a *monumentum*, a way to preserve history, which can be extended also to the built environment. See also Spencer (2007, 65).

348 See Aristodemou (2011) and Lamare (2011) on this relationship, especially, in addition to Burrell (2006, especially 457) and Rogers (2015, 355–406; 2018, 183–88).

349 Moore 1994, 15. One of Moore's more interesting water-related projects was the Piazza d'Italia in New Orleans (completed in 1978). He was also noted for collaborating with the landscape architect Laurence Halprin.

can be linked to religious practices, issues of landscape, notions of consumption, and the idea of pleasure.

6.4.1 Religion

In Book Seven of the *Aeneid*, Latinus receives a prophecy concerning the impending arrival of the Trojans and how that would affect his daughter, Lavinia (*Aen.* 7.81–84). Latinus, then, goes to the shrine of his own father, Faunus. At the shrine, which is also surrounded by a grove, the landscape resounds with the sound of a sacred spring, the *fons sacer*. Servius, writing a commentary in the fourth century CE on the *Aeneid*, felt the need to gloss this particular phrase, stating that *nullus enim fons non sacer*, that is "for there is no spring that is not sacred" (*Ad Aen.* 7.84). Whether or not water was always sacred to the Romans has been discussed since the time of the modern German scholar, Georg Wissowa.[350] It is proposed here that water was considered sacred by Romans in all contexts, given its own origins as a naturally occurring element associated with the gods.[351]

The inherent qualities of water made it a special substance vital to the religious practice of the Romans, who were by no means the only ancient peoples who revered water.[352] The purity of water was prized by the Romans, a fact that many Latin authors mention when explaining the qualities of good water. For example, Pliny the Younger describes the water associated with the shrine of the Clitumnus River as *purus et vitreus*, sparkling and clear like glass.[353] The actual or symbolic purity of water seems to be an underlying factor in the

350 Wissowa 1902, 219–25.

351 For a full discussion of these issues, see Rogers (2015, 266–354), including an overview of the cult of the Roman nymphs.

352 While there is not space in the present work for a full discussion of the religious practice of the Romans regarding water, there are a number of recent publications that can guide the reader: Seppilli 1977, 53–65; Fabre 2004; Dall'Aglio 2009; Di Giuseppe and Serlorenzi 2010; Costa, Palahí, and Vivó 2011; Calderone 2012; Giontella 2012; Rogers 2015, 266–354. De Cazanove (2015) compactly problematizes the issues of water in religious practices of the Greek and Romans. For the Greeks, see: Cole (1988) and Fenet (2016), along with Osanna (2015) for Lucanian examples. For the Etruscans and the areas that they inhabited, see: Prayon 1990; Chellini 2002, 235; Dall'Aglio 2009, 72–94. For outside of Italy, see: Alcock 1965; Krug 1985, 172–185; Green 1986, 138–62; Alarcão 1988, 102; Bourgeois 1991; Bourgeois 1992a; Burgers 2001, 5–6; Bel Faïda 2002; Arnaldi 2004; Peréx and Miró 2011; Andreu Pintado 2012; Maier 2012.

353 Plin. *Ep.* 8.8.2. For more on this passage, see especially Scheid (1996) and Lefèvre (2009, 260–72), along with Emerick (1998) on the archaeological remains of the temple described by Pliny.

reverence of the element.[354] In fact, Servius mentions that the priestesses of Vesta must collect water from the running stream outside the Porta Capena, and they must not set the vessels holding the water on the ground, lest they be contaminated (and thus made impure by the earth).[355] And thus, the pure quality of water made it an integral element in purification rites performed by the Romans, avoiding the taint of pollution.[356] In the same vein, water was used in marriage rites, purifying the bride, usually in the form of a bath.[357] The power of water, particularly in its life-giving and life-taking abilities, resonated with the Roman psyche, and, thus, played a significant role in Roman religious practice.

Archaeologically speaking, water was present in a number of different religious contexts in the Roman world. Most sacred spaces had some sort of small basin, a *delabrum*, for washing hands before entering the sanctuary.[358] Large-scale water-displays are often found at sites in the eastern half of the empire, such as the Hadrianic fountain in the Forecourt at Eleusis.[359] Source sanctuaries were popular religious sites, which allowed monumentalized veneration of water at its origins, such as at Zaghoan (Tunisia) and the recently discovered shrine at the start of the Aqua Traiana near Lake Bracciano, north of Rome.[360] While source sanctuaries are found throughout the Roman world, they are most popular in the western half of the empire (especially the northern provinces), which is also true of sites associated with healing waters.[361] Further,

354 Mazzarino 1969–1970, 643–45; Edlund-Berry 2006, 162–80; Lennon 2014, 46–7.

355 Ser. *Ad Aen.* 7.150. See also: Wissowa 1902, 180; Fantham 2012, 63. See Edlund-Berry (2006, 169) for the full bibliography of the ritual of the Vestal Virgins collecting water from the source of the Porta Capena.

356 *ThesCRA* 2.3a.IV.A (s.v., Purificazione, Romana, Mezzi impiegati nelle purificazioni, liquidi e unguenti; V. Saladino); De Cazanove 2015, 183–85. See Lennon (2012; 2014, 44–54) on the definition of pollution and the polluted, along with Fantham (2012).

357 Settis 1973, 685–689; Walker 1979, 107–122; Andò 1996; Poccetti 1996, especially 227–29; Jones 2005, 19; Giontella 2012, 191; *ThesCRA* 6.1.c.101–106, especially 106 (s.v., Mariage dans le monde romain, P. Moreau, A. Dardenay).

358 Facchinetti 2008, 47.

359 Longfellow 2012, 135–41; Rogers 2015, 300–302; Rogers forthcoming. For more on the phenomenon of water-displays at sanctuary entrances, see Rogers (2015, 296–308).

360 On Zaghoan, see Longfellow (2011, 146–47), with earlier bibliography. On the shrine associated with the Aqua Traiana, see Taylor et al. (2010).

361 Source sanctuaries typically highlight the water of the source, providing a focus for the pilgrims. This is not to be confused with a water sanctuary, which is a more general term for a sanctuary associated with water, such as thermal water. For more on this difference, see: Scheid 1991; Gros 1996, 440; Ben Abed and Scheid 2003; de Cazanove and Scheid 2003, 6. See also Bourgeois (1992b), Aupert (2012, 294–96), and De Cazanove (2015, 186–90). See

there is evidence for the display of water in structures associated with the imperial cult throughout the Roman world, such as at the sanctuary at Nîmes.[362]

The available ancient evidence supports the notion that water was always sacred throughout the Roman world, perhaps with some gradations in the perceived sacredness of the water. While all water was considered sacred, presumably some waters were 'more sacred' than others. For example, the waters collected by the Vestal Virgins at the Porta Capena stream were more obviously sacred than the waters of the Clitumnus River downstream from the shrine mentioned by Pliny where people could go swimming. But when considering the built environments that displayed water in religious spaces, the veneration of water in various forms was present everywhere in some form. Regional differences might be associated with climatic differences based on geography. For example, the prevalence of source sanctuaries in France and Germany could be attributed to the abundant number of naturally occurring springs there (in addition to the presence of older indigenous cults related to water).[363] Water played an important role in Roman religion, and the fact must be an underlying point of discussion in studies on the water culture of Roman society. Indeed, the sacred nature of water was evidently a major factor in the prominence of water usage by the Romans. Water was a life-giving element that was a gift of the gods for the benefit of humans.

6.4.2 Landscape

Landscape is crucial to understanding the water culture of any society. The notion of landscape has a myriad of definitions and implications, but simply put, it can be thought of as "the symbolic perception of [the] natural environment, [...] the way in which people read that environment for meaning."[364] While landscape is intimately tied to the environment and the idea of space or place, it is something more. Indeed, landscape "foregrounds cultural context and emphasizes the relationship between humankind, nature, and the inhabited

Rogers (2015, 308–20, 331–50) on source sanctuaries and healing sites. Of related interested is the research project *VBI AQUAE IBI SALVS*, funded by the Universidad Nacional de Educación a Distancia (UNED), under the direction of María J. Peréx, is an online atlas of medicinal water sites, healing baths, and water cult throughout the Iberian Peninsula, still under construction.

362 For more on the sanctuary at Nîmes, see: Anderson (2013, 186–90), with earlier bibliography, along with Rogers (2015, 327–30).

363 Rogers 2015, 353. On the indigenous cults of water of Roman Gaul, see the works of Bourgeois (1991; 1992a).

364 McInerney and Sluiter 2016a, 1.

world."[365] Landscape gives meaning to the natural world, which must take into account the human transformation of the existing environment.[366]

Landscape studies have risen to prominence in the field of Classics in the last few decades. Archaeology and anthropology have been instrumental in laying a strong foundation for the relationship between humans and the environments that surround them, such as cultural and natural landscapes.[367] In Classical Archaeology landscape has been integral in breaking away from the confines of the traditional text-based approaches; archaeologists are letting the material remains tell the story of past Mediterranean societies.[368] A publication of 1996, *Human Landscapes in Classical Antiquity: Environment and Culture*, was an important starting point for the discussion of landscape in antiquity, in which scholars employed a variety of evidence to understand better ancient ecology.[369] The integration of archaeological sciences with more traditional modes of historical research has helped push recent discussions about landscape in more productive directions. For example, Antonia Arnoldus-Huyzendveld, in her exploration of the landscape of the city of Rome, employs, among various approaches, climate archaeology, which has aided modern scholars in reconstructing the physicality of past landscapes.[370] In a recent Oxford University conference on fluvial landscapes new geo-archaeological methods were presented with respect to uncovering more details about the ancient climates of different rivers in the Roman world.[371] A number of scholars have explored sacred landscapes, taking the built environment and the human activities that take place there as their starting point (in lieu of explorations of the relationships between humans and nature).[372] A recent edited volume, *Valuing Landscape in Classical Antiquity: Natural Environment and Cultural Imagination*, explores landscape in the Mediterranean more fully, using a variety of philological and archaeological evidence, providing a better

365 Spencer 2010, 1.

366 Ucko and Layton 1999a, 9. See also Schama (1995, 245–306).

367 On cultural and natural landscapes, see essays in Ashmore and Knapp (1999). See the bibliography in Robinson (2016), along with Ucko and Layton (1999b), Athanassopoulos and Wandsnider (2004b), and Thomas (2006). Wylie (2007) is of particular interest.

368 See especially Athanassopoulos and Wandsnider (2004a) for a full discussion of these issues.

369 Shipley and Salmon 1996.

370 Arnoldus-Huyzendveld 2016.

371 Franconi 2017.

372 For example, see Cole (2004) and Käppel and Pothou (2015).

understanding of how ancient landscape was a cultural product of ancient Greeks and Romans.[373]

Diana Spencer has recently explored notions of Roman landscape. She demonstrates in her 2010 monograph, *Roman Landscape: Culture and Identity*, how the elements of the natural world, especially farms, gardens, and the countryside, were integral parts of what constituted being a Roman. Spencer uses theoretical models that have been prominent in a number of other disciplines (but not always in Classics), including aesthetics, hermeneutics, phenomenology, etc. While the work is short, Spencer's provocative discussions leave the reader with the desire to explore those issues more fully—hopefully inspiring further integration of new archaeological evidence to illustrate Roman landscape better.

Robinson's 2011 monograph on the Peirene spring at Corinth is an important development not only in landscape studies in the classical world, but also for water's placement in landscape. Robinson successfully demonstrates the history of the spring, from its mythological, Greek, Roman, and subsequent pasts, while stressing the importance of the water itself. The historied spring of Peirene was intimately tied to the naturally flowing waters that started high on the adjacent hill of Acrocorinth and then showed up in the city center of ancient Corinth.[374] The cultural identity that was associated with the spring, perhaps stemming from the natural hydrological landscape, was integral to Peirene's fame throughout the Greek and Roman world.[375]

Finally, Adam Rogers in his 2013 monograph, *Water and Roman Urbanism: Towns, Waterscapes, Land Transformation, and Experience in Roman Britain*, argues that water is often taken for granted in studies of ancient Roman communities. Rogers demonstrates the need for a term such as 'waterscape' that allows for the inclusion of naturally occurring water sources (for example, the economic importance of seafronts), which were integral to the culture of Roman urbanism.[376] While the research questions of Rogers are ambitious—which is to say that they are not all answered—his conception of 'waterscapes'

373 McInerney and Sluiter 2016b.

374 For more on the waters themselves, see Robinson (2011, 4–26), along with Landon (2003).

375 Robinson (2013) further explores the notions of culture and identity of Peirene and the other fountains of Corinth, especially their connections to mythological episodes, such as Bellerophon taming Pegasus at Peirene.

376 In addition to water found in terrestrial contexts, Anderson and Peters (2014) argue for exploring the human landscapes associated with the oceans of the world.

in the Roman world is crucial for better understanding Roman water culture.[377] Simply put, water was everywhere, naturally occurring, and harnessed by people. Thus, scholars must integrate this element in all of its forms as much as possible.

The notion of landscape is crucial for scholars of Roman water. While many are concerned with its final appearance and use in the built environment of the Romans, its origins in the surrounding landscape were just as important. Further, scholars can continue to explore how artificially built structures in the countryside, such as aqueducts, not only change the landscape there, but also how those structures become part of the landscape itself. Scholarship on Roman landscape has explored how Roman structures and centuriation disrupted the existing landscapes, forever altering those spaces. For example, Purcell discusses how the Roman villa, which was part of centuriation (i.e., the division and allotment of lands), began to dot the countryside, thus shaping and changing it.[378] And of the numerous activities that occurred in a rural villa or farmstead, the need of water was tantamount, meaning that with the Roman villa came water systems to supply those structures.[379] Further, Robert Witcher argues that the act of centuriation by Romans in conquered territories was an act of "physical and symbolic violence," in that "pre-existing people, places, and memories swept aside, and a new set of social relations and power asymmetries imposed on the landscape."[380] Thus, with the impostion of Roman aqueducts in the landscapes of the empire, the lives of rural residents were changed, which had positive and negative implications, ranging from the ability to have water to physical reminders of conquest.

Landscape studies concerning water in the Roman world have much to accomplish, but, with the current trends in the scholarship of Classics, perhaps more scholars will begin to integrate evidence to understand the Romans' relationship with nature. Finally, just as Robinson placed the Peirene spring in its cultural and natural landscape, scholars of Roman water must continue examining these two notions of landscape, vital to the study of Roman water usage.

6.4.3 Water's Role in Cultures of Consumption and Pleasure

Roman culture has always been noted for its embrace of pleasure. Images of hedonistic orgies and activities still remain in the popular imagination, often

377 See the review of Rippon (2014), which explores some of the problems with the monograph.

378 Purcell 1995.

379 Purcell 1995, 171.

380 Witcher 2006, 57.

in the association with the decline of Roman morals.[381] Some still believe that the *vomitorium* was a place where Romans could purge themselves of food to continue in their revelries; in reality *vomitoria* simply are the exits of Roman entertainment complexes.[382] Indeed, Roman pleasure is a nuanced subject of study. The Early empire saw a rise in pleasurable practices, and this rise has prompted scholars to analyze the so-called 'culture of consumption' popular in the Roman Empire.

Ray Laurence's 2009 monograph, *Roman Passions: A History of Pleasure in Imperial Rome*, explores the various facets of pleasure in the Roman Empire. Using different types of evidence, including literary, epigraphic, and archaeological, Laurence is able to demonstrate the nature of Roman pleasure, from private forms (e.g., food and wine consumption at a *convivium*), to more public (e.g., baths, violence in the arena), and more general forms (e.g., urban aesthetics). Laurence effectively shows that over the course of the first century CE a culture of consumption developed in Roman society, with its desire to produce new types of luxury goods and to build new environments to experience pleasure.[383]

Part of the increase in the 'pleasure culture' of Roman society was the growth of a global economy that provided more goods and technologies.[384] As other scholars have demonstrated, new building construction technologies impacted the Roman economy, with new types of building materials available through the open frontiers of the empire.[385] Thus, the new construction abilities allowed for grander architectural forms that could cater to tastes that craved newer forms of pleasure. Andrew Wallace-Hadrill has also shown the role luxuries played in the Roman world, which caused a consumer revolution, but also brought the ire of Roman orators and writers in the first century BCE.[386] The growth of the Roman economy in the first two centuries CE was driven by "a desire within Roman society to buy into a culture of pleasure, in which those who could build, consumed and magnanimously gave money to enable

381 See Wallace-Hadrill's discussion (2008, 315–29).

382 The *vomitorium* as a vaulted passageway in the Roman theater and amphitheater is found in Macrobius (*Sat.* 6.4); see also Sear (2006, 6).

383 Laurence 2009, 158–59.

384 The notion of globalization has become popular in Roman studies in the last decade, such as with Hingley (2005) and De Angelis (2013). See also the collection of essays by Pitts and Versluys (2015) that offers new perspectives on the subject, along with a response by Van Oyen (2015).

385 Saller 2002; DeLaine 2006; Wilson 2006; Laurence 2009, 158–60.

386 Wallace-Hadrill 2008, 315–55.

the masses to experience pleasure."[387] Roman pleasure reached its apex in the second century CE, but declined by the fourth century.[388] By the height of the empire, a multi-directional web of influence between pleasure, materials and technology, and economy had developed in the Roman world—all of which allowed for the experience of pleasure in various forms.

Roman uses of water fit well into a culture of pleasure. As has been alluded to throughout this discussion, Romans relished the pleasure of water. First and foremost to consider is the response to water by the five senses.[389] As already mentioned, Vitruvius reminds his reader that water was essential not only for daily survival, but also pleasure (*De arch.* 8.1.1). Pliny the Younger's letter to Domitius Apollinaris, which documents the amenities of Pliny's Tuscan villa, catalogues the water features therein (*Ep.* 5.6). He even describes an ornamental pool inside the villa as *strepitu visuque iucunda*, "a pleasure to hear and to see" (5.6.23).[390] Water, from its inherent physical properties, has the ability to delight and provide pleasure.

Pleasure of water also has the power to create sensory responses when added to man-made constructions, such as in baths or water-displays. In the case of the imperial *thermae* of Rome, resplendent with flowing water, grand architecture, and exotic decorations, the sensory experience of the bathing ritual was a *tour de force*.[391] The water in the baths was also transformative physically and psychologically. The water itself in the rooms in and around the *caldarium* would have turned to steam. And the heat of the steam not only caused bathers to relax, but also dulled the senses, as vision in particular is hindered in a room full of steam. Moreover, the pleasure associated with water in the baths could also be extended to the activities that took place in those spaces, from relaxation to sexual adventures.[392] Thus, while water can be a pleasure in and of itself, it is water's ability to alter physical spaces—and one's own sensory perceptions—that contributed to the 'pleasure culture' of Roman society.

---

387 Laurence 2009, 162.

388 Laurence 2009, 162.

389 For an overview of ancient Roman responses to water using the five senses, see Rogers (2015, 105–28). On sensory experiences in Roman culture, see Toner (2014) and Betts (2017), which builds upon a growing trend in sensory studies related to the ancient world, such as the work of Hamilakis (2014). For more on the connections between Roman water-displays and sensory responses, see Rogers (2015; forthcoming).

390 Rogers 2013, 155; Rogers 2015, 94–105.

391 Yegül 2010, 6, 126–32.

392 On the same-sex sexual activities that took place in the Roman bath-house, see the article of Eger (2007), who compares the Roman baths with modern gay bath houses with great success. See also Laurence's discussion (2009, 63–74), based on Eger's arguments.

Romans' 'culture of pleasure' prompted changes in the architecture of water-related structures. Seneca the Younger in *Letter* 56 laments how bathing complexes have changed from the austere structures of the time of Scipio Africanus to Seneca's own day in the first century CE. With some panache, Seneca describes the new baths:

> Pauper sibi videtur ac sordidus nisi parietes magnis et pretiosis orbibus refulserunt, nisi Alexandrina marmora Numidicis crustis distincta sunt, nisi illis undique operosa et in picturae modum variata circumlitio praetexitur, nisi vitro absconditur camera, nisi Thasius lapis, quondam rarum in aliquo spectaculum templo, piscinas nostras circumdedit, in quas multa sudatione corpora exsaniata demittimus, nisi aquam argentea epitonia fuderunt. Et adhuc plebeias fistulas loquor: quid cum ad balnea libertinorum pervenero? Quantum statuarum, quantum columnarum est nihil sustinentium sed in ornamentum positarum impensae causa! quantum aquarum per gradus cum fragore labentium! Eo deliciarum pervenimus ut nisi gemmas calcare nolimus.
>
> *EP.* 86.6–7

> But who in these days could bear to bathe in such a fashion [as Scipio]? We think ourselves poor and mean if our walls are not resplendent with large and costly mirrors; if our marbles from Alexandria are not set off by mosaics of Numidian stone, if their borders are not faced over on all sides with difficult patterns, arranged in many colors like paintings; if our vaulted ceilings are not buried in glass; if our swimming-pools are not lined with Thasian marble, once a rare and wonderful sight in any temple—pools into which we let down our bodies after they have been drained weak by abundant perspiration; and finally, if the water has not poured from silver spigots. I have so far been speaking of the ordinary bathing-establishments; what shall I say when I come to those of the freedmen? What a vast number of statues, of columns that support nothing, but are built for decoration, merely in order to spend money! And what masses of water that fall crashing from level to level! We have become so luxurious that we will have nothing but precious stones to walk upon.
>
> TRANS. R.M. GUMMERE

In addition to the presence of exotic marbles and statues, Seneca states that the vaulted ceilings can accommodate windows, which allow sunlight to penetrate the baths.[393] Further, there is an abundance of water flowing in the baths, 'crashing from level to level,' which certainly changed its physical appearance as it flowed down each level, while at the same time the sound of its movement filled the space with noise. Again, the insatiable culture of consumption in the first and second centuries CE of the empire fueled the popularity of water structures and the many pleasures that they afforded, like bath-houses.[394] Bruun has recently argued that the display of water in public baths was the only time that ancient writers could attack the luxurious use of water, especially because it could lead to other unsavory behaviors in the baths.[395] The growth of the empire, from its frontiers, to its economy, to advances in building technology, only allowed for a greater exploitation by Romans of the pleasurable qualities of water, despite continued moral attacks.

While water has important life-giving qualities that Romans depended on for survival, because of the vast resources available to the state, the more pleasurable, luxurious aspects of water were also showcased throughout the empire. Indeed, pleasure transcends utility. With new ways to construct physical environments, Romans created novel and spectacular methods for using and displaying water. Although these constructions often served utilitarian purposes, the collective desire to experience the pleasures of water in a variety of contexts prompted the proliferation of water structures across the Mediterranean during the High Roman Empire. Thus, Roman pleasure culture played a significant role in the development of empire-wide trends in building and using water structures; this phenomenon is integral to understanding the complex nature of Roman water culture.

7 Conclusions

The culture of water in Roman society was pervasive, but malleable. The dissemination of water technologies allowed for the growth of cities throughout the empire, no matter their location, since large urban centers are

393 For more on windows, especially at the Baths of Carcalla, see Yegül (2010, 113). On the practice of Roman sunbathing, see Zarmakoupi (2014, 163–74).

394 Laurence 2009, 66.

395 Bruun 2016a. In his article, Bruun argues that while Latin writers were castigating private luxuries, private water use in the city of Rome was not attacked, as private water rights were tied to an imperial benefaction (and thus to the emperor himself). It was only the public baths of the era that led to moralistic admonitions.

unsustainable without a sufficient and reliable water source.[396] Again, Roman water culture was not monolithic, meaning that, while there was a common, inherent need to have water and a desire to use and to display it in some way, different communities throughout the empire used water-related structures of varying degrees of scale and complexity.

A notion of adaptive water culture strongly parallels current arguments regarding the conception of Roman identity. Over the last two decades, scholars have begun to demonstrate the nuances of Roman identity throughout the empire—namely that it was "dynamic, continually evolving, and changing."[397] For example, Amanda Kelly has shown how Roman bathhouses on Crete are a mixture of Roman and indigenous elements, demonstrating how a population can still craft their own identity, while also exhibiting identifiable Roman traits.[398] Paolo Vitti has shown how vaulting techniques in the Peloponnese incorporated not only technology from Rome and Northern Italy, but also local techniques, creating a unique type of vaulting (using more bricks and less concrete mortar) that was employed in structures like aqueducts and fountains.[399] Roman identity is not straightforward, and it is unfair to prescribe a blanket culture of water for all of the inhabitants of the vast empire. But throughout the Roman world, elements of Roman water culture were employed to varying degrees, which helped to tie the various peoples of the empire together. Water, regardless of its context, helps to establish, foster, and reinforce communal senses of identity.[400] Thus, water culture is an important avenue of investigation for understanding better the other cultural, social, political, and economic aspects of Roman life.

The work of many of the scholars presented here has helped to discern avenues of further inquiry into Roman water culture. As Hodge prescribed in 1991, the future currents of the field should include the better integration of technology and engineering studies with historical explorations of Roman water structures. To a certain extent, this is being achieved by meetings of the Frontinus Gesellschaft and other scholars, such as Richard (2012). In the same

396 Wilson 2012, 3.

397 Mattingly 2004, 10. The scholarship related to Roman identity is ever-growing and naturally complex. For more, see the discussions in Revell (2009; 2016) and in the edited volume of Gardner, Herring, and Lomas (2013). Revell also explores the notions of 'ethnic identities' in the Roman Empire (2016, 19–39).

398 Kelly 2013.

399 Vitti 2016.

400 Ceccarelli 2012, 1.

vein, scholars are beginning to study water systems more holistically, highlighting where water comes from, how it arrives in an urban setting, and how it is consumed. New evidence, especially when approached with new methodologies and archaeological technologies, has allowed scholars to rethink canonical elements of Roman water culture. Lead poisoning and ancient issues of hygiene are at the forefront of this discussion.

There is still more to be done, however. The field would benefit from larger diachronic and regional studies to provide a more complete understanding of just how water was sourced, collected, and used. But this is, naturally, a difficult task, not only due to the extent of the empire and its centuries of water usage, but also the available evidence, which is so expansive that it is almost impossible to synthesize fully. The goal of this contribution was to illustrate some of the most important issues facing scholars concerning the perception, use, and enjoyment of water during the Roman period. Water had an enormous impact on the growth and success of the empire; even after its collapse, Roman methods of exploiting water were continued by subsequent peoples—demonstrating the social and cultural importance of water in all time periods. By studying water in the Roman world, scholars can better understand other related elements of Roman culture, allowing for more nuanced discussions of the Romans themselves, and their relationships with other groups of people, let alone nature itself.

References

Abadie-Reynal, Catherine, Samuel Provost, and Pascal Vipard, eds. 2011. *Les réseaux d'eau courante dans l'antiquité: Réparations, modifications, réutilisations, abandon, récupération*. Renne: Presses Universitaires de Rennes.

Agusta-Boularot, Sandrine. 1997. "La fontaine, la ville et le Prince. Recherches sur les fontaines monumentales et leur fonction dans l'urbanisme impérial, de l'avénement d'Auguste au règne des Sévères." Ph.D. diss., Université de Provence, Aix-Marseille 1.

Agusta-Boularot, Sandrine. 2001. "Fontaines et fontaines monumentales en Grèce de la conquête romaine à l'époque Flavienne: Permanence ou renouveau architectural?" In *Constructions publiques et programmes édilitaires en Grèce entre le IIe siècle av. J.-C. et le Ier siècle ap. J.-C.*, edited by Jean-Yves Marc and Jean-Charles Moretti, 167–236. *BCH* Suppl. 39. Paris: De Boccard.

Agusta-Boularot, Sandrine. 2004. "Les fontaines urbaines en Gaule." In *Fontaines et Nymphées en Gaule Romaine: Fontaines publiques et privées, les nymphées dans les thermes*, edited by S. Agusta-Boularot and Éric Follain, 4–11. Les Dossiers d'Archeologie 295. Dijon: Éditions Faton.

Agusta-Boularot, Sandrine. 2008. "Le *lacus* de la rue romaine: Un exemple de 'mobilier urbain' antique?" In *La rue dans l'Antiquité: Définition, aménagement et devenir*, edited by Pascale Ballet et al., 93–100. Rennes: Presses Universitaires de Rennes.

Agusta-Boularot, Sandrine, and Éric Follain, eds. 2004. *Fontaines et Nymphées en Gaule Romaine: Fontaines publiques et privées, les nymphées dans les thermes*. Les Dossiers d'Archeologie 295. Dijon: Éditions Faton.

Aicher, Peter J. 1995. *Guide to the Aqueducts of Ancient Rome*. Wauconda, IL: Bolchazy-Carducci.

Alarcão, Jorge. 1988. *Roman Portugal*. Warminster, England: Aris & Phillips, Ltd.

Alcock, Joan P. 1965. "Celtic Water Cults in Roman Britain." *AJ* 122: 1–12.

Alcock, Susan E. 1995. "Pausanias and the *Polis*: Use and Abuse." In *Sources for the Ancient Greek City-State, Acts of the Copenhagen Polis Centre, Vol. 2*, edited by Mogens H. Hansen, 326–44. Copenhagen: Munksgaard.

Aldrete, Gregory S. 2007. *Floods of the Tiber in Ancient Rome*. Baltimore: Johns Hopkins University Press.

Ambrogi, Annarena. 2005. Labra *di età romana in marmi bianchi e colorati*. Studia Archeologia 136. Rome: "L'Erma" di Bretschneider.

Amit, David, Joseph Patrich, and Yizhar Hirschfeld, eds. 2002. *The Aqueducts of Israel*. *JRA* Suppl. 46. Portsmouth, RI: JRA.

Anderson, James C. 2013. *Roman Architecture in Provence*. Cambridge: Cambridge University Press.

Anderson, James C. 2014. "Architect and Patron." In *A Companion on Roman Architecture*, edited by Roger B. Ulrich and Caroline K. Quenemoen, 127–39. Malden, MA: Wiley-Blackwell.

Anderson, Jon, and Kimberley Peters. 2014. "'A Perfect and Absolute Blank': Human Geographies of Water World." In *Water Worlds: Human Geographies of the Ocean*, edited by J. Anderson and K. Peters, 3–19. Farnham: Ashgate.

Andò, Valeria. 1996. "*Nymphe*: la sposa e le ninfe." *QUCC* 52.1: 47–79.

Andreu Pintado, Javier. 2012. "Aspectos sociales del culto a las aguas en *Hispania*: las dedicaciones a las *Nymphae*." In *L'eau: usages, risques et répresentations dans le Soud-Ouest de la Gaule et le Nord de la péninsule Ibérique, da la fin de l'âge du Fer à l'Antiquité tardive* (*II*[e] *s. a.C.–VI*[e] *s. p.C.*), edited by Jean-Pierre Bost, 333–47. Aquitania Suppl. 21. Bordeaux: Aquitania.

Aristodemou, Georgia. 2011. "Theatre Façades and the Façade Nymphaeum. The Link Between." *BCH* 135: 163–97.

Aristodemou, Georgia. 2012. *Ο Γλυπτός Διάκοσμος Νυμφαίων και Κρηνών, στο Ανατολικό Τμήμα της Ρωμαϊκής Αυτοκρατορίας* [*Sculptured Decoration of Monumental Nymphaea and Fountains at the Eastern Provinces of the Roman Empire*]. Thessaloniki: Κορνηλία Σφακιανάκη.

Aristodemou, Georgia, and Theodosios P. Tassios, eds. 2018. *Great Waterworks of Roman Greece: Aqueducts and Monumental Fountains, Function in Context*. Oxford: Archaeopress.

Arnaldi, Adelina. 2004. "Osservazioni sul culto delle Nymphae nell'Africa romana." In *L'Africa romana: Ai confini dell'impero; Contatti, scambi, conflitti; Atti del XV Convegno di studio (Tozeur, 11–15 dicembre 2002)*, edited by Mustapha Khanoussi, 1355–64. Rome: Carocci.

Arnoldus-Huyzendveld, Antonia. 2016. "Aspects of the Landscape Environment of Rome in Antiquity: Changes of Landscape, Shift of Ideas." In *Le regole del gioco: Tracce, archeologi, racconti: Studi in onore di Clemetina Panella*, edited by Antonio F. Ferrandes and Giacomo Pardini, 177–202. LTUR Suppl. 6. Rome: Edizioni Quasar.

Arvanitis, Nikoloas. 2008. *I tiranni e le acque: Infrastrutture idrauliche e potere nella Grecia del tardo arcaismo*. Bologna: D.u. Press.

Ashby, Thomas. 1935. *The Aqueducts of Ancient Rome*. Oxford: Clarendon Press.

Ashmore, Wendy, and A. Bernard Knapp, eds. 1999. *Archaeologies of Landscape*. Oxford: Blackwell.

Athanassopoulos, Effie-Fotini, and LuAnn Wandsnider. 2004a. "Mediterranean Landscape Archaeology Past and Present." In *Mediterranean Archaeological Landscapes: Current Issues*, edited by E.-F. Athanassopoulos and L. Wandsnider, 1–14. Philadelphia: University of Pennsylvania Museum of Archaeology and Anthropology.

Athanassopoulos, Effie-Fotini, and LuAnn Wandsnider, eds. 2004b. *Mediterranean Archaeological Landscapes: Current Issues*. Philadelphia: University of Pennsylvania Museum of Archaeology and Anthropology.

Aubert, Jean-Jacques. 1994. *Business Managers in Ancient Rome: A Social and Economic Study of* Institores, *200 B.C.–200 A.D.* Leiden: Brill.

Aupert, Pierre. 1974. *Le nymphée de Tipasa et les nymphées et "septizonia" nord-africains*. Collection de l'École Française de Rome 16. Rome: École Française de Rome.

Aupert, Pierre. 2012. "Eau et religion." In *L'eau: usages, risques et représentations dans le Sud-Ouest de la Gaule et le Nord de la péninsule Ibérique de la fin de l'age du Fer à l'Antiquité tardive (IIe s. a.C.–VIe s. p.C.)*, edited by Jean-Pierre Bost, 293–320. Aquitania Suppl. 21. Bordeaux: Aquitania.

Balty, Jean-Charles. 1962. "Vestiges de robinetterie romaine." *Revue Archéologique de l'Est et du Centre-Est* 13: 277–88.

Bannon, Cynthia J. 2001. "Servitudes for Water Use in the Roman *Suburbium*." *Historia* 50.1: 34–52.

Bannon, Cynthia J. 2009. *Gardens and Neighbors: Private Water Rights in Roman Italy*. Ann Arbor: University of Michigan Press.

Bannon, Cynthia J. 2013. "Pipes and Property in the Sale of Real Estate (D.19.1.38.2)." In *New Frontiers: Law and Society in the Roman World*, edited by Paul J. Du Plessis, 207–23. Edinburgh: Edinburgh University Press.

Barker, Graeme, and David Gilbertson, eds. 2000. *The Archaeology of Drylands: Living at the Margin*. London: Routledge.

Bartsch, Shadi. 1994. *Actors in the Audience: Theatricality and Doublespeak from Nero to Hadrian*. Cambridge, MA: Harvard University Press.

Beacham, Richard C. 1991. *The Roman Theatre and its Audience*. London: Routledge.

Beacham, Richard C. 1999. *Spectacle Entertainments of Early Imperial Rome*. New Haven: Yale University Press.

Bedon, Robert, ed. 1997. *Les aqueducs de la Gaule romaine et des regions voisines*. Limoges: Punim.

Behr, Charles A. 1981. *P. Aelius Aristides. The Complete Works: vol. 2: Orations XVII–LIII*. Leiden: Brill.

Bel Faïda, Abdelaziz. 2002. "Eau et sacré en Afrique romaine." *L'Africa romana* 14: 1715–28.

Bell, Andrew. 2004. *Spectacular Power in the Greek and Roman City*. Oxford: Oxford University Press.

Bell, Malcolm. 1994. "An Imperial Flour Mill on the Janiculum." In *La ravitaillement en blé de Rome et des centres urbains des débuts de la République jusqu'au Haut Empire*, [no ed.], 73–89. Collection de l'École Française de Rome 196. Rome: École Française de Rome.

Beltrán Lloris, Francisco. 2006. "An Irrigation Decree from Roman Spain: the *Lex rivi Hiberiensis*." *JRS* 96: 147–97.

Ben Abed, Aïcha, and John Scheid. 2003. "Sanctuaire des eaux, sanctuaire de sources, une catégorie ambiguë: l'exemple de Jebel Oust (Tunisie)." In *Sanctuaires et sources dans l'Antiquité: Les sources documentaires et leurs limites dans la description des lieux de culte*, edited by Olivier de Cazenove and J. Scheid, 7–14. Collection du Centre Jean Bérard 22. Naples: Centre Jean Bérard.

Berg, Deena. 1994. "Fountains and Artistic Water Displays in Classical Antiquity: Origins and Development from 700 to 30 B.C." Ph.D. diss., University of Texas at Austin.

Berlan-Bajard, Anne. 2006. *Les spectacles aquatiques Romains*. Collection de l'École Française de Rome 360. Rome: École Française de Rome.

Berno, Francesca R. 2012. "Non solo acqua. Elementi per un diluvio universale nel terzo libro delle *Naturales Quaestiones*." In *Seneca e le scienze naturali*, edited by Marco Beretta et al., 69–80. Florence: Leo S. Olschki Editore.

Betts, Eleanor, ed. 2017. *Senses of the Empire: Multisensory Approaches to Roman Culture*. London: Routledge.

Bianchi, Elisabetta, ed. 2015. *La Cloaca Maxima e i sistemi fognari di Roma dall'antichità ad oggi*. Rome: Palombi Editori.

Bianco, Anna D. 2007. Aqua ducta, aqua distributa*: La gestione delle risorse idriche in età romana*. Torino: Silvio Zamorani Editore.

Black, Maggie. 2016. *The Atlas of Water: Mapping the World's Most Critical Resource*. 3rd ed. Oakland: University of California Press.

Blackman, Deane R., and A. Trevor Hodge. 2001. *Frontinus' Legacy: Essays on Frontinus'* De Aquis Urbis Romae. Ann Arbor: University of Michigan Press.

Blonski, Michel. 2014. *Se nettoyer à Rome (IIe siècle av. J.-C.–IIe siècle ap. J.-C.): Pratiques et enjeux*. Paris: Les Belles Lettres.

Blyth, P.H. 1999. "The Consumption and Cost of Fuel in Hypocaust Baths." In *Roman Baths and Bathing: Proceedings of the First International Conference on Roman Baths held at Bath, England, 30 March–4 April 1992*, edited by Janet DeLaine and David E. Johnson, 87–98. Portsmouth, RI: JRA.

Bodin, Helena. 2016. "'Rejoice, Spring': The Theotokos as Fountain in the Liturgical Practice of Byzantine Hymnography." In *Fountains and Water Culture in Byzantium*, edited by Brooke Shilling and Paul Stephenson, 229–45. Cambridge: Cambridge University Press.

Bol, Renate. 1984. *Das Statuenprogramm des Herodes-Atticus-Nymphäums. Olympische Forschungen* 15. Berlin: Walter de Gruyter.

Bonneau, Danielle. 1964. *La crue du Nile, divinité Égyptienne à travers mille ans d'histoire (332 av.–641 ap. J.-C.)*. Paris: Klincksieck.

Bonneau, Danielle. 1993. *Le régime administrative de l'eau du Nil dans l'Égypte grecque, romaine et byzantine*. Leiden: Brill.

Boucher, Jean-Paul, ed. 1983. *Journées d'études sur les aqueducs romains. Tagung über römische Wasserversorgungsanlagen, Lyon, 26–28 mai, 1977*. Paris: Les Belles Lettres.

Bourgeois, Claude. 1991. *Divona I: Divinités et ex-voto du culte gallo-romain de l'eau*. Paris: De Boccard.

Bourgeois, Claude. 1992a. *Divona II: Monuments et sanctuaires du culte gallo-romain de l'eau*. Paris: De Boccard.

Bourgeois, Claude. 1992b. "L'aménagement des sanctuaires de l'eau." In *Dieux guérisseurs en Gaule romaine*, edited by Christian Landes, 21–4. Lattes: Musée Archéologique Henri Prades.

Boussac, Marie-Françoise, Thibaud Fournet, and Bérangère Redon, eds. 2009. *Le bain collectif en Égypte*. Cairo: Institut français d'archeologie orientale.

Braconi, Paolo, ed. 2013. *Il santuario di Diana a Nemi: Le terrazze e il ninfeo, Scavi 1989–2009*. Studia Archeologia 194. Rome: "L'Erma" di Bretschneider.

Bressan, Marianna. 2003. "I ninfei." In Subterraneae Domus*: Ambienti residenziali e di servizio nell'edilizia privata romana*, edited by Patrizia Basso and Francesca Ghedini, 235–301. Sottosuolo del Mondo Antico 4. Caselle di Sommacampagna: Cierre Edizioni.

Brinker, Werner. 1990. *Wasserspeicherung in Zisternen: Ein Beitrag zur Frage der Wasserversorgung früher Städte*. Braunschweig: Leichtweiss-Institut für Wasserbau.

Brun, Jean-Pierre. 2007. "L'énergie hydraulique durant l'empire romain: Quel impact sur l'économie agricole?" In *Innovazione tecnica e progresso economico nel mondo romano*, edited by Elio Lo Casio, 101–103. Bari: Edipuglia.

Brun, Jean-Pierre, and Jean-Luc. Fiches, eds. 2007. *Énergie hydraulique et machines élévatrices d'eau dans l'antiquité*. Paris: De Boccard.

Bruun, Christer. 1991. *The Water Supply of Ancient Rome: A Study in Roman Imperial Administration*. Helsinki: Societas Scientiarum Fennica.

Bruun, Christer. 1992. "Water as a Cruel Element in the Roman World." In *Crudelitas: The Politics of Cruelty in the Ancient and Medieval World*, edited by Toivo Viljamaa, Asko Timonen, and Christian Krötzl, 74–80. Krems: Medium Aevum Quotidianum.

Bruun, Christer. 2000. "Water Legislation in the Ancient World (c. 2200 B.C.–c. A.D. 500)." In *Handbook of Ancient Water Technology*, edited by Örjan Wikander, 539–604. Technology and Change in History 2. Leiden: Brill.

Bruun, Christer. 2001. "Imperial Water Pipes in Roman Cities." In *Water Use and Hydraulics in the Roman City*, edited by Ann Olga Koloski-Ostrow, 51–64. Dubuque, IA: Kendall/Hunt Publishing.

Bruun, Christer. 2003. "Frontinus and the "Nachleben" of his *De aquaeductu* from Antiquity to the Baroque." In *Technology, Ideology, Water: From Frontinus to the Renaissance and Beyond*, edited by C. Bruun and Ari Saastamoinen, 41–80. Rome: Institutum Romanum Finlandiae.

Bruun, Christer. 2007. "*Aquaeductium* e *statio aquarum*. La sede della *cura aquarum* di Roma." In Res bene gestae: *Ricerche di storia urbana su Roma antica in onore di Eva Margareta Steinby*, edited by Anna Maria Leone, Domenico Palombi, and Susan Walker, 1–13. Rome: Edizioni Quasar.

Bruun, Christer. 2010. "*Instrumentum domesticum* e storia romana: Le fistule iscritte della Campania." In *Il Mediterraneo e la storia. Epigrafia e archeologia in Campania: letture storiche*, edited by Laura Chioffi, 145–83. Naples: Luciano Editore.

Bruun, Christer. 2012a. "Cola di Rienzo and the Lost Clause on Changing the Course of Rivers in the *Lex de imperio Vespasiani*." In *Per una comune cultura dell'acqua. Dal Mediterraneo all'America del Nord*, edited by Fara Nasti and Francesca Reduzzi Merola, 109–34. Cassino: Università degli Studi di Cassino e del Lazio Meridionale.

Bruun, Christer. 2012b. "New Prosopographical Data Derived from Roman Lead Pipe Inscriptions." *Arctos* 46: 19–31.

Bruun, Christer. 2012c. "Roman Emperors and Legislation on Public Water Use in the Roman Empire: Clarifications and Problems." *Water History* 4.1: 11–33.

Bruun, Christer. 2012d. "Stallianus, a Plumber from Pompeii (and Other Remarks on Pompeian Lead Pipes)." *Phoenix* 66.1–2: 145–47.

Bruun, Christer. 2015a. "Gaetano Marini studioso delle *fistulae aquariae* romane." In *Gaetano Marini (1742–1815) protagonista della cultura europea. Scritti per il bicentenario della morte*, [no ed.], 1017–37. Rome: Vatican.

Bruun, Christer. 2015b. "Water Use and Productivity in Roman Agriculture: Selling, Sharing, Servitudes." In *Ownership and Exploitation of Land and Natural Resources in the Roman World*, edited by Paul Erdkamp, Koenraad Verboven, and Arjan Zuiderhoek, 132–51. Oxford: Oxford University Press.

Bruun, Christer. 2016a. "L'acqua come elemento di lusso nella cultura romana: da Varrone alla *Historia Augusta*." *MEFRA* (online) 128.1. [DOI: 10.4000/mefra.3250].

Bruun, Christer. 2016b. "Inscriptions on Roman Water Pipes: A Global Survey." In *De aquaeductu atque aqua urbium Lyciae Pamphyliae Pisidiae: The Legacy of Sextus Julius Frontinus*, edited by Gilbert Wiplinger, 9–22. *BABesch* Suppl. 27. Leuven: Peeters.

Bukowiecki, Évelyne, Hélène Dessales, and Julien Dublouloz. 2008. *Ostie, l'eau dans la ville: Châteaux d'eau et réseau d'adduction*. Rome: École Française de Rome.

Burgers, Alfonso. 2001. *The Water Supplies and Related Structures of Roman Britain*. British Archaeological Reports-British Series 324. Oxford: Archaeopress.

Burrell, Barbara. 2006. "False Fronts: Separating the Aedicular Façade from the Imperial Cult in Roman Asia Minor." *AJA* 110.3: 437–69.

Burrell, B. 2012. "Book Review of *Roman Imperialism and Civic Patronage: Form, Meaning, and Ideology in Monumental Fountain Complexes*." *AJA* 116.2 (online). [https://www.ajaonline.org/book-review/1107]. (Last accessed 13 September 2017)

Busch, Stephan. 1999. *Versus Balnearum: Die antike Dichtung über Bäder und Baden im römischen Reich*. Stuttgart: B.G. Teubner.

Calderone, Anna, ed. 2012. *Cultura e religione dell'acqua: atti del Convegno interdisciplinare "Qui fresca l'acqua mormora ..." (S. Quasimodo, Sapph. fr. 2,5)*. Rome: Giorgio Bretschneider Editore.

Camardo, Domenico, Monica Martelli Castaldi, and Jane Thompson. 2006. "Water Supply and Drainage at Herculaneum." In *Cura Aquarum in Ephesus*, vol. 2, edited by Gilbert Wiplinger, 183–91. *BABesch* Suppl. 12. Leuven: Peeters.

Camp, John M. 1991. "Water Supply and its Historical Context." In *Future Currents in Aqueduct Studies*, edited by A. Trevor Hodge, 105–11. Leeds: Francis Cairns.

Campagna, Lorenzo. 2011. "Le fontane nella città dell'impero romano: 'Monuments Indelibly Associated with the Emperor'?" *JRA* 24: 648–56.

Campbell, Brian. 2012. *Rivers and the Power of Ancient Rome*. Chapel Hill: University of North Carolina Press.

Cariou, Gérald. 2009. *La Naumachie: Morituri te salutant*. Paris: Presses de l'université Paris-Sorbonne.

Ceccarelli, Paola. 2012. "Water and Identity in the Ancient Mediterranean." *MHR* 27.1: 1–3.

Chellini, Riccardo. 2002. *Acque sorgive salutari e sacre in Etruria (Italiae Regio VII): Ricerche archaeologiche e di topografia antica*. British Archaeological Reports-International Series 1067. Oxford: Archaeopress.

Chi, Jennifer. 2002. "Studies in the Programmatic Statuary of Roman Asia Minor." Ph.D. diss., New York University.

Chirassi Colombo, Ileana. 2004. "Figure d'acqua: Albunea, Mefitis e la Sibilla tiburtina." In *Acque per l'utilitas, per la salubritas, per l'amoenitas*, edited by Mariavittoria Antico Gallina, 299–316. Milan: ET.

Christaki, Maria, George K. Stournaras, Panagiotis T. Nastos, Nikos Mamassis. 2017a. "Water Supply Associated with the Development of the City of Athens from the Hellenistic Era until the End of the Nineteenth Century." *Water History* 9.4: 389–410 [https://doi.org/10.1007/s12685-017-0198-x].

Christaki, Maria, George K. Stournaras, Panagiotis T. Nastos, Nikos Mamassis. 2017b. "Water Supply Associated with the Development of the City of Athens from the End of the Nineteenth Century until the Present." *Water History* 9.4: 411–31 [https://doi.org/10.1007/s12685-017-0197-y].

Cilliers, Louise. 1993. "Public Health in Roman Legislation." *AClass* 36: 1–10.

Cochet, André. 2000. *Le plomb en Gaule romaine. Techniques de fabrication et produits*. Montagnac: Edition M. Mergoil.

Cole, Susan Gettel. 1988. "The Uses of Water in Greek Sanctuaries." In *Early Greek Cult Practice: Proceedings of the Fifth International Symposium at the Swedish Institute in Athens, 26–29 June 1986*, edited by Robin Hägg, Nanno Marinatos, and Gullög C. Nordquist, 161–65. Stockholm: Paul Åstöms Förlag.

Cole, Susan Gettel. 2004. *Landscapes, Gender, and Ritual Space: The Ancient Greek Experience*. Berkeley: University of California Press.

Coleman, Kathleen M. 1993. "Launching into History: Aquatic Display in the Early Empire." *JRS* 83: 48–74.

Coleman, Kathleen M. 2006. "BMCR Review of Andrew Bell, *Spectacular Power in the Greek and Roman City*." *BMCRev* 2006.04.04. [http://bmcr.brynmawr.edu/2006/2006-04-04.html]. (Last accessed 13 September 2017)

Coleman, Kathleen M. 2008. "'Not Waving but Drowning': Total Immersion in Aquatic Displays." *JRA* 21.2: 458–64.

Coleman, Kathleen M., ed. 2014. *Le jardin dans l'antiquité*. Entretiens sur l'antiquité classique 60. Geneva: Fondation Hardt.

Confronto, Maria L. 1991. "Terme di Caracalla: Dati acquisiti ed ipotesi di ricerca." In *Les Thermes Romains: Actes de la table ronde organisée par l'École Française de Rome (Rome, 11–12 novembre 1988)*, edited by René Rebuffat, 43–8. Portsmouth, RI: JRA.

Costa, Ana, Luís Palahí, and David Vivó, eds. 2011. *Aquae Sacrae: Agua y sacralidad en la Antigüedad*. Girona: Institut de Recerca Històrica de la Universitat de Girona.

Crouch, Dora. 1993. *Water Management in Ancient Greek Cities*. Oxford: Oxford University Press.

Crouch, Dora. 2003. *Geology and Settlement: Greco-Roman Patterns*. Oxford: Oxford University Press.

Crow, James. 2012a. "Ruling the Waters: Managing the Water Supply of Constantinople, A.D. 330–1204." *Water History* 4.1: 35–55.

Crow, James. 2012b. "Water and Late Antique Constantinople: 'It Would be Abominable for the Inhabitants of this Beautiful City to be Compelled to Purchase Water.'" In *Two Romes: Rome and Constantinople in Late Antiquity*, edited by Lucy Grig and Gavin Kelly, 116–35. Oxford: Oxford University Press.

Crow, James, Jonathan Bardill, and Richard Bayliss. 2008. *The Water Supply of Byzantine Constantinople*. JRS Monograph No. 11. London: Society for the Promotion of Roman Studies.

Cunliffe, Barry W. 1995. *Roman Bath*. London: B.T. Batsford.

Curd, Patricia, and Daniel W. Graham. 2008. *The Oxford Handbook of Presocratic Philosophy*. Oxford: Oxford University Press.

Dall'Aglio, Michele. 2009. *I culti delle acque nell'Italia Antica*. Imola: Angelini Editore.

D'Arms, John. 1999. "Performing Culture: Roman Spectacle and the Banquets of the Powerful." In *The Art of Ancient Spectacle*, edited by Bettina Bergmann and Christine Kondoleon, 301–19. Studies in the History of Art 56. Washington: National Gallery of Art.

Dauterman Maguire, Eunice. 2016. "Spouts and Finials Defining Fountains by Giving Water Shape and Sound." In *Fountains and Water Culture in Byzantium*, edited by Brooke Shilling and Paul Stephenson, 163–81. Cambridge: Cambridge University Press.

Davies, Alison E. 1997. "The Role of Inscribed Monuments in Transforming Public Space at Pompeii and Ostia." D.Phil. thesis, University of Oxford.

Day, Jo. 2017. "Scents of Place and Colours of Smell: Fragranced Entertainment in Ancient Rome." In *Senses of the Empire: Multisensory Approaches to Roman Culture*, edited by Eleanor Betts, 176–92. London: Routledge.

De Angelis, Franco, ed. 2013. *Regionalism and Globalism in Antiquity: Exploring their Limits*. Leuven: Peeters.

De Cazanove, Olivier. 2015. "WATER." In *A Companion to the Archaeology of Religion in the Ancient World*, edited by Rubina Raja and Jörg Rüpke, 181–93. Chichester: Wiley Blackwell.

De Cazanove, Olivier, and John Scheid, eds. 2003. *Sanctuaires et sources dans l'Antiquité: Les sources documentaries et leurs limites dans la description des lieux de culte*. Naples: Centre Jean Bérard.

De Haan, Nathalie. 2010. *Römische Privatbäder: Entwicklung, Verbreitung, Struktur und sozialer Status*. Frankfurt am Main: Peter Lang.

De Kleijn, Gerda. 2001. *The Water Supply of Ancient Rome: City Area, Water, and Population*. Amsterdam: J.C. Gieben.

De Kleijn, Gerda. 2016. "*Fistulae* and Water Fraud in Late Antique Constantinople." In *Fountains and Water Culture in Byzantium*, edited by Brooke Shilling and Paul Stephenson, 36–54. Cambridge: Cambridge University Press.

DeLaine, Janet. 1996. "'*De aquis suis*'?: The "*Commentarius*" of Frontinus." In *Les littératures techniques dans l'antiquité romaine: Statut, public et destination, tradition*, edited by Claude Nicolet and Pierre Gros, 117–45. Geneva: Vandoevres.

DeLaine, Janet. 1997. *The Baths of Caracalla: A Study in Design, Construction, and Economics of Large-Scale Building Projects in Imperial Rome*. Portsmouth, RI: JRA.

DeLaine, Janet. 2006. "The Cost of Creation: Technology at the Service of Construction." In *Innovazione tecnica e progresso economico nel mondo romano*, edited by Elio Lo Casio, 237–52. Bari: Edipuglia.

Del Chicca, Fanny. 1997. "Terminologia delle fontane publiche a Roma: *lacus, salientes, munera*." *RCCM* 39: 231–53.

Del Chicca, Fanny. 2004. *Frontino,* De Aquae Ductu Urbis Romae*: Introduzione, testo critico, traduzione e commento*. Rome: Herder Editrice e Libreria.

Delile, Hugo, Janne Bilchert-Toft, Jean-Philippe Goiran, Simon Keay, and Francis Albarède. 2014. "Lead in Ancient Rome's City Waters." *Proceedings of the National Academy of Sciences of the United States of America* 111.18: 6594–99.

De Robertis, Francesco M. 1936. *La espropriazione per pubblica utilità nel diritto romano*. Bari: Pubblicazioni dell'Istituto di diritto romano della R. Università di Bari.

Dessales, Hélène. 2013. *Le partage de l'eau: Fontaines et distribution hydraulique dans l'habitat urbain de l'Italie romaine*. Bibliothèque des Écoles Françaises d'Athènes et de Rome 351. Rome: École Française de Rome.

Di Giuseppe, Helga, and Mirella Serlorenzi, eds. 2010. *I riti del costruire nelle acque violate*. Rome: Scienze e Lettere, Bardi Editore.

Donahue, John F. 2015. "The Healing Springs of Latium and Etruria." In *Aspects of Ancient Institutions and Geography: Studies in Honor of Richard J.A. Talbert*, edited by Lee L. Brice and Daniëlle Slootjes, 314–32. Leiden: Brill.

Dorl-Klingenschmid, Claudia. 2001. *Prunkbrunnen in kleinasiatischen Städten: Funktion im Kontext*. München: Verlag Dr. Friedrich Pfeil.

Dorl-Klingenschmid, Claudia. 2006. "Brunnenbauten als Medium des interkommunalen Wettbewerbs." In *Cura Aquarum in Ephesus*, vol. 2, edited by Gilbert Wiplinger, 381–86. *BABesch* Suppl. 12. Leuven: Peeters.

Drogula, Fred K. 2000. "The Curule Aedileship and the Conception of Office in Republican Rome." MA thesis, University of Virginia.

Dupré Raventós, Xavier, and Joseph Anton Remolà Vallverdú, eds. 2000. Sordes Urbis: *La eliminación de residuos en la ciudad romana*. Rome: "L'Erma" di Bretschneider.

Eck, Werner. 1987. "Die Wasserversorgung im römischen Reich: Sozio-politische Bedingungen, Recht und Administration." In *Die Wasserversorgung antiker Städte. Pergamon. Recht/Verwaltung. Brunnen/Nymphäen. Bauelemente*, [no ed.], 49–101. *Geschichte der Wasserversorgung* 2. Mainz: Verlag Philip von Zabern.

Eck, Werner. 1998. "Die *fistulae aquariae* der Stadt Rom. Zum Einfluß des sozialen Status auf administratives Handeln." In *Die Verwaltung des römischen Reiches in der Hohen Kaiserzeit: ausgewählte und erweiterte Beiträge Bd.* 2, edited by W. Eck, 245–77. Basel: Reinhardt.

Edlund-Berry, Ingrid. 2006. "Hot, Cold, or Smelly: The Power of Sacred Water in Roman Religion, 400–100 BCE." In *Religion in Republican Italy*, edited by Celia E. Schultz and Paul B. Harvey, 162–80. *YClS* Suppl. 33. Cambridge: Cambridge University Press.

Edmondson, Jonathan C. 1999. "The Cultural Politics of Public Spectacle in Rome and the Greek East, 167–166 BCE." In *The Art of Ancient Spectacle*, edited by Bettina Bergmann and Christine Kondoleon, 77–95. Studies in the History of Art 56. Washington: National Gallery of Art.

Eger, A. Asa. 2007. "Age and Male Sexuality: 'Queer Space' in the Roman Bath-House?" In *Age and Ageing in the Roman Empire*, edited by Mary Harlow and Ray Laurence, 131–51. Portsmouth, RI: JRA.

Ehrlich, Tracy L. 1989. "The Waterworks of Hadrian's Villa." *The Journal of Garden History* 9.4: 161–76.

Ellis, S.P. 1997. "Pooling Resources: The Use of Water for Social Control in the Roman Empire." In *TRAC 96: Proceedings of the Sixth Annual Theoretical Roman Archaeology Conference*, edited by Karen Meadows et al., 144–50. Oxford: Oxbow Books.

Emerick, Judson J. 1998. *The Tempietto del Clitumno near Spoleto*. University Park, PA: Pennsylvania State University Press.

Evans, Harry B. 1993. "*In Tiburtium usum*: Special Arrangements in the Roman Water System (Frontinus, *Aq.* 6.5)." *AJA* 97.3: 447–55.

Evans, Harry B. 1997. *Water Distribution in Ancient Rome: The Evidence of Frontinus*. Ann Arbor: University of Michigan Press.

Fabre, Guilhem. 2004. "Divinidades y cultos relacionados con las aguas." In *Aqua Romana: Tècnica humana i força divina*, [no ed.], 146–61. Barcelona: Fundación Agbar.

Fabre, Guilhem, Jean-Luc Fiches, and Jean-Louis Paillet, ed. 2000. *L'aqueduc de Nîmes et le Pont du Gard: archéologie, géosytème, histoire*. 2nd ed. Paris: CNRS Éditions.

Facchinetti, Grazia. 2008. "Offrire nelle acque: Bacini e altre strutture artificiali." In *I riti del costruire nelle acque violate*, edited by Helga di Giuseppe and Mirella Serlorenzi, 43–67. Rome: Scienze e Lettere, Bardi Editore.

Fagan, Garrett G. 1999. *Bathing in Public in the Roman World*. Ann Arbor: University of Michigan Press.

Fagan, Garrett G. 2000. "Hygienic Conditions in Roman Public Baths." In *Cura Aquarum in Sicilia*, edited by Gemma C.M. Jansen, 281–87. *BABesch* Suppl. 6. Leiden: Peeters.

Fagan, Garrett G. 2001. "The Genesis of the Roman Public Bath: Recent Approaches and Future Directions." *AJA* 105.3: 403–26.

Fahlbusch, Henning, ed. 2008. *Die Wasserkultur der Villa Hadriana*. Norderstedt: Books on Demand.

Fantham, Elaine. 2012. "Purification in Ancient Rome." In *Rome, Pollution, and Propriety: Dirt, Disease, and Hygiene in the Eternal City from Antiquity to Modernity*, edited by Mark Bradley, 59–66. Cambridge: Cambridge University Press.

Farrar, Linda. 1998. *Ancient Roman Gardens*. Stroud: Stroud Publishing.

Farrar, Linda. 2016. *Gardens and Gardeners of the Ancient World: History, Myth, and Archaeology*. Oxford: Windgather Press.

Farrington, Andrew. 1995. *The Roman Baths of Lycia: An Architectural Study*. London: British Institute of Archaeology at Ankara.

Favro, Diane. 1999. "The City Is a Living Thing: The Performative Role of an Urban Site in Ancient Rome, the Vallis Murcia." In *The Art of Ancient Spectacle*, edited by Bettina Bergmann and Christine Kondoleon, 205–19. Studies in the History of Art 56. Washington: National Gallery of Art.

Feldherr, Andrew. 1998. *Spectacle and Society in Livy's* History. Berkeley: University of California Press.

Fenet, Annick. 2016. *Les dieux olympiens et la mer: espaces et pratiques cultuelles*. Rome: École Française de Rome.

Fernández Casado, Carlos. 1972. *Acueductos romanos en España*. Madrid: Instituto Eduardo Torroja.

Fevrier, Paul-Albert. 1983. "Armée et aqueducts." In *Journées d'études sur les aqueducs romains. Tagung über römische Wasserversorgungsanlagen, Lyon, 26–28 mai, 1977*, edited by Jean-Paul Boucher, 133–40. Paris: Les Belles Lettres.

Fleury, Philippe. 2005. "La pompe à pistons dans l'Antiquité." In Aquam in altum exprimere: *Les machines élévatrices d'eau dans l'Antiquité*, edited by Alain Bouet, 139–52. Scripta Antiqua 12. Pessac: Ausonius Éditions.

Fleury, Philippe. 2008a. "La *machina Ctesibica*. Comment projeter de l'eau sous pression dans l'Antiquité?" In *Archéologie et histoire des techniques du monde romain*, edited by Michel Molin, 119–32. Paris: De Boccard.

Fleury, Philippe. 2008b. "Les *sparsiones* liquides dans les spectacles romains." *REL* 86: 97–112.

Flohr, Miko. 2011. "The Uses and Value of Urine." In *Roman Toilets: Their Archaeology and Cultural History*, edited by Gemma C.M. Jansen, Ann Olga Koloski-Ostrow, and Eric M. Moorman, 149–54. *BABesch* Suppl. 19. Leuven: Peeters

Fournet, Thibaud, and Bérangère Redon. 2013. "Heating Systems of Greek Baths: New Evidence from Egypt." In *Greek Baths and Bathing Culture: New Discoveries and Approaches*, edited by Sandra K. Lucore and Monika Trümper, 239–63. *BABesch* Suppl. 23. Leuven: Peeters.

Franconi, Tyler V., ed. 2017. *Fluvial Landscapes in the Roman World*. *JRA* Suppl. 104. Portsmouth, RI: JRA.

Garbrecht, Günther. 2001. *Stadt und Landschaft: Teil 4, Die Wasserversorgung von Pergamon*. Berlin: Walter de Gruyter.

Gardner, Andrew, Edward Herring, and Kathryn Lomas, eds. 2013. *Creating Ethnicities & Identities in the Roman World*. BICS 120. London: Institute of Classical Studies.

Gauly, Bardo M. 2004. *Senecas* Naturales Quaestiones*: Naturphilosophie für die römische Kaiserzeit*. Munich: Verlag C.H. Beck.

Gensheimer, Maryl B. Forthcoming. *Decoration and Display in Rome's Imperial Thermae: Messages of Power and their Popular Reception at the Baths of Caracalla*. Oxford: Oxford University Press.

Geremia Nucci, Roberta. 2001. "Les *fistulae aquariae* inscrites d'Ostie." In *Ostia: Port et porte de la Rome antique*, edited by Jean-Paul Descoeudres, 108–13. Chêne-Bourg: Georg.

Geremia Nucci, Roberta. 2006. "I *plumbarii* ostensi: una sintesi delle nuove evidenze." *ArchClass* 57: 447–67.

Gibson, Roy K., and Ruth Morello., eds. 2011. *Pliny the Elder: Themes and Contexts*. *Mnemosyne* Suppl. 329. Leiden: Brill.

Gilfillan, S. Colum. 1965. "Lead Poisoning and the Fall of Rome." *Journal of Occupational Medicine* 7: 53–60.

Ginouvès, René. 1962. *Balaneutikè: Recherches sur le bain dans l'antiquité grecque*. Paris: Éditions E. de Boccard.

Ginouvès, René. 1969. "L'Architecture." In *Laodicée du Lycos: Le Nymphée, Campagnes 1961–1963*, edited by Jean Des Gagniers et al., 13–185. Recherches Archéologiques, Série 1. Québec: Presses de l'Université Laval.

Giontella, Claudia. 2012. "… Nullus enim fons non sacer …": *Culti idrici di epoca preromana e romana (Regiones VI–VII)*. Pisa: Fabrizio Serra Editore.

Giorgi, Elisabetta. 2007. "Water Technology at Gortyn in the 4th–7th C. A.D.: Transport, Storage, and Distribution." In *Technology in Transition A.D. 300–650*, edited by Luke Lavan, Enrico Zanini, and Alexander C. Sarantis, 287–320. Late Antique Archaeology 6. Leiden: Brill.

Giorgi, Elisabetta. 2016. *Archeologia dell'acqua a Gortina di Creta in età protobizantina*. Oxford: Archeopress.

Glaser, Franz. 1983. *Antike Brunnenbauten (KRHNAI) in Griechenland*. Wien: Verlag der Österreichischen Akademie der Wissenshaften.

Gleason, Kathryn, ed. 2013. *A Cultural History of Gardens in Antiquity*. London: Bloomsbury.

González Soutelo, Silvia. 2012. "Thermal Spas in the Roman Age: An Approximation to the Architectonic Configuration of Baths with Mineral-Medicinal Water in Hispania." In *SPA, Sanitas per Aquam: Proceedings of the International Frontinus-Symposium on the Technical and Cultural History of Ancient Baths*, edited by Ralf Kreiner and Wolfram Letzner, 79–86. *BABesch* Suppl. 21. Leuven: Peeters.

Gowers, Emily. 1995. "The Anatomy of Rome from Capitol to Cloaca." *JRS* 85: 23–32.

Green, Miranda. 1986. *The Gods of the Celts*. Brigdend: Sutton.

Greene, Kevin. 1994. "Technology and Innovation in Context: The Roman Background to Medieval and Later Developments." *JRA* 7: 22–33.

Grewe, Klaus. 1986. *Atlas der römischen Wasserleitungen nach Köln*. Rheinischen Ausgrabungen 26. Köln: Rheinland Verlag.

Grewe, Klaus. 1998. *Licht am Ende des Tunnels: Planung und Trassierung im antiken Tunnelbau*. Mainz am Rhein: Verlag Philipp von Zabern.

Grewe, Klaus. 2008. "Tunnels and Canals." In *The Oxford Handbook of Engineering and Technology in the Classical World*, edited by John Peter Oleson, 319–36. Oxford: Oxford University Press.

Grewe, Klaus. 2016. *Aquädukte: Wasser für Roms Städte, der große Überblick, vom Römerkanal zum Aquäducktmarmor*. Rheinbach: Regionalia Verlag.

Grig, Lucy, and Gavin Kelly. 2012. "Introduction: From Rome to Constantinople." In *Two Romes: Rome and Constantinople in Late Antiquity*, edited by L. Grig and G. Kelly, 3–30. Oxford: Oxford University Press.

Gros, Pierre. 1996. *L'architecture romaine du debut du IIIe siècle av. J.-C. à la fin du Haut-Empire: Vol. 1, Les monuments publics*. Paris: Picard.

Gross, Nikolaus. 1989. *Senecas* Naturales Quaestiones: *Komposition, naturphilosophische Aussagen und ihre Quellen*. Stuttgart: Franz Steiner Verlag.

Hamilakis, Yannis. 2014. *Archaeology and the Senses: Human Experience, Memory, and Affect*. Cambridge: Cambridge University Press.

Healy, John F. 1999. *Pliny the Elder on Science and Technology*. Oxford: Oxford University Press.

Heller, Anna. 2006. *'Les bêtises des Grecs.' Conflicts et rivalités entre cités d'Asie et de Bithynie à l'époque romaine (129 a.C.–235 p.C.)*. Scripta Antiqua 17. Bordeaux: Ausonius Éditions.

Hermon, Ella, ed. 2008. *Vers une gestion intégrée de l'eau dans l'empire romain*. Rome: "L'Erma" di Bretschneider.

Hermon, Ella, ed. 2010. Riparia *dans l'empire romain: pour la définition du concept*. British Archaeological Reports-International Series 2066. Oxford: British Archaeological Reports.

Hine, Harry M. 2010. *Seneca: Natural Questions, The Complete Works of Lucius Anneaus Seneca*. Chicago: University of Chicago Press.

Hingley, Richard. 2005. *Globalizing Roman Culture: Unity, Diversity and Empire*. London: Routledge.

Hobson, Barry. 2009a. Latrinae et Foricae: *Toilets in the Roman World*. London: Duckworth.

Hobson, Barry. 2009b. *Pompeii, Latrines and Down Pipes: A General Discussion and Photographic Record of Toilet Facilities in Pompeii*. British Archaeological Reports-International Series 2041. Oxford: British Archaeological Reports.

Hodge, A. Trevor. 1991. "Conclusion." In *Future Currents in Aqueduct Studies*, edited by A.T. Hodge, 163–74. Leeds: Francis Cairns.

Hodge, A. Trevor. 1992. *Roman Aqueducts and Water Supply*. London: Duckworth.

Hodge, A. Trevor. 2000a. "Aqueducts." In *Handbook of Ancient Water Technology*, edited by Örjan Wikander, 39–66. Technology and Change in History 2. Leiden: Brill.

Hodge, A. Trevor. 2000b. "Qanats." In *Handbook of Ancient Water Technology*, edited by Örjan Wikander, 35–8. Technology and Change in History 2. Leiden: Brill.

Hodge, A. Trevor. 2000c. "Wells." In *Handbook of Ancient Water Technology*, edited by Örjan Wikander, 29–34. Technology and Change in History 2. Leiden: Brill.

Hodge, A. Trevor. 2002. *Roman Aqueducts and Water Supply*. 2nd ed. London: Duckworth.

Hopkins, John N. 2007. "The Cloaca Maxima and the Monumental Manipulation of Water in Archaic Rome." *Waters of Rome* 4. [www3.iath.virginia.edu/waters/Journal4Hopkins.pdf]. (Last accessed 13 September 2017)

Hopkins, John N. 2012. "The 'Sacred Sewer': Tradition and Religion in the Cloaca Maxima." In *Rome, Pollution, and Propriety: Dirt, Disease, and Hygiene in the Eternal City from Antiquity to Modernity*, edited by Mark Bradley, 81–102. Cambridge: Cambridge University Press.

Jackson, Ralph. 1999. "Spas, Waters, and Hydrotherapy in the Roman World." In *Roman Baths and Bathing: Proceedings of the First International Conference on Roman Baths held at Bath, England, 30 March–4 April 1992*, edited by Janet DeLaine and David E. Johnson, 107–16. Portsmouth, RI: JRA.

Jacobs, Ine, and Julian Richard. 2012. "'We Surpass the Beautiful Waters of Other Cities by the Abundance of Ours': Reconciling Function and Decoration in Late Antique Fountains." *Journal of Late Antiquity* 5.1: 3–71.

Jansen, Gemma C.M. 2000a. "Studying Roman Hygiene: the Battle between the 'Optimists' and the 'Pessimists.'" In *Cura Aquarum in Sicilia*, edited by G.C.M. Jansen, 275–79. *BABesch* Suppl. 6. Leiden: Peeters.

Jansen, Gemma C.M. 2000b. "Systems for the Disposal of Waste and Excreta in Roman Cities: The Situation in Pompeii, Herculaneum, and Ostia." In *Sordes Urbis: La eliminación de residuos en la ciudad romana*, edited by Xavier Dupré Raventós and Joseph Anton Remolà Vallverdú, 37–49. Rome: "L'Erma" di Bretschneider.

Jansen, Gemma C.M. 2000c. "Urban Water Transport and Distribution." In *Handbook of Ancient Water Technology*, edited by Örjan Wikander, 103–25. Technology and Change in History 2. Leiden: Brill.

Jansen, Gemma C.M. 2001. "Water Pipe Systems in the Houses of Pompeii: Distribution and Use." In *Water Use and Hydraulics in the Roman City*, edited by Ann Olga Koloski-Ostrow, 27–40. Dubuque, IA: Kendall/Hunt Publishing.

Jansen, Gemma C.M. 2003. "Social Distinctions and Issues of Privacy in the Toilets of Hadrian's Villa." *JRA* 16.1: 137–52.

Jansen, Gemma C.M., Ann Olga Koloski-Ostrow, and Eric M. Moorman. 2011a. "Introduction." In *Roman Toilets: Their Archaeology and Cultural History*, edited by G.C.M. Jansen, A.O. Koloski-Ostrow, and E.M. Moorman, 1–5. *BABesch* Suppl. 19. Leuven: Peeters.

Jansen, Gemma C.M., Ann Olga Koloski-Ostrow, and Eric M. Moorman, eds. 2011b. *Roman Toilets: Their Archaeology and Cultural History*. *BABesch* Suppl. 19. Leuven: Peeters.

Jashemski, Wilhelmina F. 1979. *The Gardens of Pompeii: Herculaneum and the Villas Destroyed by Vesuvius*. New Rochelle, NY: Caratzas Brothers Publishers.

Jashemski, Wilhelmina F., Kathryn L. Gleason, Kim J. Hartswick, and Amina-Aïcha Malek, eds. 2017. *Gardens of the Roman Empire*. Cambridge: Cambridge University Press.

Jenewein, Gunhild. 2008. *Die Architekturdekoration der Caracallathermen*. Wien: Verlag der Östereichischen Akademie der Wissenschaften.

Jones, Christopher P. 1991. "Aelius Aristides. 'On the Water in Pergamon.'" *AA* 111–17.

Jones, Prudence J. 2005. *Reading Rivers in Roman Literature and Culture*. New York: Lexington Books.

Jones, Rick, and Damian Robinson. 2005. "Water, Wealth, and Social Status at Pompeii: The House of the Vestals in the First Century." *AJA* 109.4: 695–710.

Kamash, Zena. 2008. "What Lies Beneath? Perceptions of the Ontological Paradox of Water." *World Archaeology* 40.2: 224–37.

Kamash, Zena. 2010. *Archaeologies of Water in the Roman Near East*. Piscataway, NJ: Gorgias Press.

Kamash, Zena. 2012. "An Exploration of the Relationship between Shifting Power, Changing Behaviour and New Water Technologies in the Roman Near East." *Water History* 4.1: 79–93.

Kapossy, Balázs. 1969. *Brunnenfiguren der hellenistischen und römischen Zeit*. Zürich: Juris Druck & Verlag.

Käppel, Lutz, and Vassiliki Pothou, eds. 2015. *Human Development in Sacred Landscapes*. Goettingen: VetR unipress.

Keenan-Jones, Duncan C. 2016. "Fountains, Lead Pipes and Water Systems in Pompeii, Rome, and the Roman West." *JRA* 29.2: 778–85.

Keenan-Jones, Duncan C., John Hellstrom, and Russell Drysdale. 2011. "Lead Contamination in the Drinking Water of Pompeii." In *Pompeii: Art, Industry, and Infrastructure*, edited by Eric Poehler, Miko Flohr, and Kevin Cole, 131–48. Oxford: Oxbow Books.

Kehoe, Dennis. 2008. "Economics and the Law of Water Rights in the Roman Empire." In *Vers une gestion intégrée de l'eau dans l'empire romain*, edited by Ella Hermon, 243–51. Rome: "L'Erma" di Bretschneider.

Kek, Damir. 1996. *Der römische Aquädukt als Bautypus und Repräsentationsarchitektur.* Münster: Charybdis.

Kellum, Barbara. 1999. "The Spectacle of the Street." In *The Art of Ancient Spectacle*, edited by Bettina Bergmann and Christine Kondoleon, 283–99. Studies in the History of Art 56. Washington: National Gallery of Art.

Kelly, Amanda. 2013. "Roman Bathhouses on Crete as Indicators of Cultural Transition: The Dynamics of Roman Influence." In *Creating Ethnicities & Identities in the Roman World*, edited by Andrew Gardner, Edward Herring, and Kathryn Lomas, 131–68. *BICS* 120. London: Institute of Classical Studies.

Kimmelfield, Isabel. 2016. "The Shrine of the Theotokos at the Pege." In *Fountains and Water Culture in Byzantium*, edited by Brooke Shilling and Paul Stephenson, 281–98. Cambridge: Cambridge University Press.

Kleiner, Fred S. 1991. "The Trophy on the Bridge and the Roman Triumph over Nature." *AC* 60: 182–92.

Köhler, Jens. 2012. "Death in the Bath: From Therapeutic Hazard to a Reconstruction of Ancient Roman Bathing." In *SPA, Sanitas per Aquam: Proceedings of the International Frontinus-Symposium on the Technical and Cultural History of Ancient Baths*, edited by Ralf Kreiner and Wolfram Letzner, 191–202. *BABesch* Suppl. 21. Leuven: Peeters.

Köhler, Jens. 2016. "Der hadrianische und antoninische Değirmendere Aquädukt von Ephesos: 10 Jahre nach dem Ephesos-Symposium." In *De aquaeductu atque aqua urbium Lyciae Pamphyliae Pisidiae: The Legacy of Sextus Julius Frontinus*, edited by Gilbert Wiplinger, 55–64. *BABesch* Suppl. 27. Leuven: Peeters.

Koloski-Ostrow, Ann Olga. 2001. "Water as a Symbol of Wealth? An Overview of the Roman Evidence." In *Water Use and Hydraulics in the Roman City*, edited by A.O. Koloski-Ostrow, 1–15. Dubuque, IA: Kendall/Hunt Publishing.

Koloski-Ostrow, Ann Olga. 2008. "Water, water (literally) everywhere: Turkey, Italy, Greece, Near East, & Mesopotamia, N Africa, Gallia, Germania, Spain." *JRA* 21.2: 549–56.

Koloski-Ostrow, Ann Olga. 2015a. *The Archaeology of Sanitation in Roman Italy: Toilets, Sewers, and Water Systems*. Chapel Hill: University of North Carolina Press.

Koloski-Ostrow, Ann Olga. 2015b. "Urban Smells: Archaeological Evidence." In *Smell and the Ancient Senses*, edited by Mark Bradley, 90–109. London: Routledge.

Koloski-Ostrow, Ann Olga, Nathalie de Haan, Gerda de Kleijn, and Susanna A.G. Piras. 1997. "Water in the Roman Town: New Research from *Cura Aquarum* and the *Frontinus Society*." *JRA* 10: 181–91.

Koloski-Ostrow, Ann Olga, and Steven E. Ostrow. 2014. "New Approaches to Urban Sanitation, Pollution, and Propriety in *Hispania* and for the City of Rome." *JRA* 27.2: 578–83.

Kondoleon, Christine. 1999. "Timing Spectacles: Roman Domestic Art and Performance." In *The Art of Ancient Spectacle*, edited by Bettina Bergmann and C. Kondoleon, 321–41. Studies in the History of Art 56. Washington: National Gallery of Art.

Kreiner, Ralf, and Wolfram Letzner, eds. 2012. *SPA, Sanitas per Aquam: Proceedings of the International Frontinus-Symposium on the Technical and Cultural History of Ancient Baths. BABesch* Suppl. 21. Leuven: Peeters.

Kretzschmer, Fritz. 1960. "La robinetterie romaine." *Revue Archéologique de l'Est et du Centre-Est* 11: 89–113.

Krug, Antje. 1985. *Heilkunst und Heilkult: Medizin in der Antike*. München: Verlag C.H. Beck.

Kuhn, Christina T. 2013. "Der Rangstreit der Städte im römischer Kleinasien: Anmerkungen zu Kontext und Datierung von *I.Laodikeia* 10." *ZPE* 186: 195–204.

Kullberg, Jesper B. 2016. "When Bath Became Church: Spatial Fusion in Late Antique Constantinople and Beyond." In *Fountains and Water Culture in Byzantium*, edited by Brooke Shilling and Paul Stephenson, 130–44. Cambridge: Cambridge University Press.

Kuttner, Ann. 1999. "Hellenistic Images of Spectacle, from Alexander to Augustus." In *The Art of Ancient Spectacle*, edited by Bettina Bergmann and Christine Kondoleon, 97–123. Studies in the History of Art 56. Washington: National Gallery of Art.

Lamare, Nicolas. 2011. "L'influence de l'architecture théâtrale dur le décor des fontaines monumentales." In *Le passé et son heritage: Modalités et enjeux dans les sociétés du monde romain et de l'Antiquité tardive*, edited by N. Lamare et al., 28–45. Paris: "Orient et Méditerranée."

Lamare, Nicolas. 2014. "Les fontaines monumentales en Afrique romaine." Ph.D. diss., Université Paris-Sorbonne.

Landon, Mark E. 2003. "Beyond Peirene: Toward a Broader View of Corinthian Water Supply." In *Corinth, The Centenary, 1896–1996*, edited by Charles K. Williams and Nancy Bookidis, 43–62. *Corinth* 20. Princeton: American School of Classical Studies at Athens.

Laurence, Ray. 2009. *Roman Passions: A History of Pleasure in Imperial Rome*. London: Continuum.

Lavagne, Henri. 1990. "Fontane e ninfei." In *Civiltà dei Romani: La città, il territorio, l'impero*, edited by Salvatore Settis, 125–38. Naples: Electa.

Lavagne, Henri. 1992. "Le problème des 'Nymphées' en Gaul." In *Les eaux thermales et les cultes des eaux: en Gaule et dans les provinces voisines*, edited by Raymond Chevallier, 217–25. Tours: Centre de Recherches A. Piganiol.

Lavagne, Henri. 2012. "Quelques fontaines publiques et nymphées en Gaule romaine." In *L'eau en Méditerranée de l'Antiquité au Moyen Âge*, edited by Jacques Jouanna et al., 117–39. Cahiers de la Villa Kérylos 23. Paris: De Broccard.

Lebel, Paul. 1965. "Vestiges de robinetterie Romaine." *Revue Archéologique de l'Est et du Centre-Est* 16: 259–73.

Lefèvre, Eckard. 2009. *Vom Römertum zum Ästhetizismus: Studien zu den Briefen des jüngeren Plinius*. Berlin: Walter de Gruyter.

Lehar, Hannes. 2012. *Die römische Hypokaustheizung: Berechnungen und Überlegungen zu Leistung, Aufbau und Funktion*. Aachen: Shaker Verlag.

Leigh, Shawna. 1997. "The 'Reservoir' of Hadrian in Athens." *JRA* 10: 279–90.

Leigh, Shawna. 1998. "The Aqueduct of Hadrian and the Water Supply of Roman Athens." Ph.D. diss., University of Pennsylvania.

Leigh, Shawna. 2001. "A Survey of the Early Roman Hydraulics in Athens." In *Water Use and Hydraulics in the Roman City*, edited by Ann Olga Koloski-Ostrow, 65–82. Dubuque, IA: Kendall/Hunt Publishing.

Lendon, Jon E. 2015. "Rhetoric and Nymphaea in the Roman Empire." *Chiron* 45: 123–45.

Lennon, Jack J. 2012. "Pollution, Religion, and Society in the Roman World." In *Rome, Pollution, and Propriety: Dirt, Disease, and Hygiene in the Eternal City from Antiquity to Modernity*, edited by Mark Bradley, 43–58. Cambridge: Cambridge University Press.

Lennon, Jack J. 2014. *Pollution and Religion in Ancient Rome*. Cambridge: Cambridge University Press.

Lessler, Milton A. 1988. "Lead and Lead Poisoning from Antiquity to Modern Times." *Ohio Journal of Science* 88.3: 78–84.

Letzner, Wolfram. 1990. *Römische Brunnen und Nymphaea in der westlichen Reichschälfte*. Münster: Charybdis.

Letzner, Wolfram. 1999. *Römische Brunnen und Nymphaea in der westlichen Reichschälfte*. 2nd Rev. Ed. Münster: Charybdis.

Letzner, Wolfram. 2013. "Zur Terminologie römische Brunnenanlagen." In *Die Wasserversorgung im antiken Rom Sextus Iulius Frontinus, sein Werk in lateinisch und Deutsch und begleitende Fachaufsätze*, [no ed.], 231–42. *Geschichte der Wasserversorgung* 2, 2nd ed. München DIV Deutscher Industrieverlag.

Leveau, Philippe. 1991. "Research on Roman Aqueducts in the Past Ten Years." In *Future Currents in Aqueduct Studies*, edited by A. Trevor Hodge, 149–62. Leeds: Francis Cairns.

Leveau, Philippe. 1996. "The Barbegal Water Mill and its Environment: Archaeology and the Economic and Social History of Antiquity." *JRA* 9: 137–53.

Leveau, Philippe. 2007. "Les moulins de Barbegal, 1986–2006." In *Énergie hydraulique et machines élévatrices d'eau dans l'antiquité*, edited by Jean-Pierre Brun and Jean-Luc Fiches, 185–99. Paris: De Boccard.

Lewis, Michael J.T. 1999. "Vitruvius and Greek Aqueducts." *PBSR* 67: 145–72.

Lewis, Michael J.T. 2000. "Theoretical Hydraulics, Automata, and Water Clocks." In *Handbook of Ancient Water Technology*, edited by Örjan Wikander, 343–69. Technology and Change in History 2. Leiden: Brill.

Lewis, Michael J.T. 2007. "Antique Engineering in the Byzantine World." In *Technology in Transition A.D. 300–650*, edited by Luke Lavan, Enrico Zanini, and Alexander C. Sarantis, 367–78. Late Antique Archaeology 6. Leiden: Brill.

Liverani, Mario, ed. 2003. *Arid Lands in Roman Times*. Arid Zone Archaeology Monographs 4. Florence: Edizioni all'Insegna del Giglio.

Longfellow, Brenda. 2010. "Reflections of Imperialism: The Meta Sudans in Rome and the Provinces." *The Art Bulletin* 92.4: 275–92.

Longfellow, Brenda. 2011. *Roman Imperialism and Civic Patronage: Form, Meaning, and Ideology in Monumental Fountain Complexes*. Cambridge: Cambridge University Press.

Longfellow, Brenda. 2012. "Roman Fountains in Greek Sanctuaries." *AJA* 116: 133–55.

Longfellow, Brenda. 2016. "The Silahtarağa Statues in Context." In *Fountains and Water Culture in Byzantium*, edited by Brooke Shilling and Paul Stephenson, 55–67. Cambridge: Cambridge University Press.

Longfellow, Brenda. 2018. "Reflecting the Past: The Nymphaeum Near the So-Called Praetorium at Gortyn." In *Great Waterworks of Roman Greece: Aqueducts and Monumental Fountains, Function in Context*, edited by Georgia Aristodemou and Theodosios P. Tassios, 246–58. Oxford: Archaeopress.

Louis, Pierre. 1982. "L'eau et sa legislation chez Platon et Aristotle." In *L'Homme et l'eau en Méditerranée et au Proche Orient, 2*, edited by Françoise Métral and Jean Métral, 103–10. Lyon: Presses Universitaires.

Lucore, Sandra K. 2013. "Bathing in Hieronian Sicily." In *Greek Baths and Bathing Culture: New Discoveries and Approaches*, edited by S.K. Lucore and Monika Trümper, 151–80. *BABesch* Suppl. 23. Leuven: Peeters.

Lucore, Sandra K. 2016. "Greek Baths." In *A Companion to Greek Architecture*, edited by Margaret M. Miles, 328–41. Malden, MA: Wiley Blackwell.

Lucore, Sandra K., and Monika Trümper, eds. 2013. *Greek Baths and Bathing Culture: New Discoveries and Approaches*. *BABesch* Suppl. 23. Leuven: Peeters.

Lusnia, Susann. 2004. "Urban Planning and Sculptural Display in Severan Rome: Reconstructing the Septizodium and its Role in Dynastic Politics." *AJA* 108: 517–44.

Lytle, Beth G. 2015. "Water, *Aemulatio*, and Legitimization: Republican and Early Augustan Fountains in the City of Rome." Ph.D. diss., Emory University.

MacDonald, William L., and John A. Pinto. 1995. *Hadrian's Villa and its Legacy*. New Haven: Yale University Press.

Magdalino, Paul. 2016. "The Culture of Water in the 'Macedonian Renaissance.'" In *Fountains and Water Culture in Byzantium*, edited by Brooke Shilling and Paul Stephenson, 103–29. Cambridge: Cambridge University Press.

Maier, Bernhard. 2012. *Geschichte und Kultur der Kelten*. München: Verlag C.H. Beck.

Malissard, Alain. 1994. *Les Romains et l'Eau: Fontaines, salles de bains, themes, égouts, aqueducs*. Paris: Les Belles Lettres.

Manderscheid, Hubertus. 1991. "La gestione idrica delle Terme di Caracalla: Alcune osservazioni." In *Les Thermes Romains: Actes de la table ronde organisée par l'École Française de Rome (Rome, 11–12 novembre 1988)*, edited by René Rebuffat, 49–60. Portsmouth, RI: JRA.

Manderscheid, Hubertus. 2000a. "The Water Management of Greek and Roman Baths." *In Handbook of Ancient Water Technology*, edited by Örjan Wikander, 467–535. Technology and Change in History 2. Leiden: Brill.

Manderscheid, Hubertus. 2000b. "Überlegungen zur Wasserarchitektur und ihrer Funktion in der Villa Adriana." *Römische Mitteilungen* 107: 109–40.

Manderscheid, Hubertus. 2002. "L'architettura dell'acqua a Villa Adriana con particolare riguardo al Canopo." In *Villa Adriana: Paesaggio antico e ambiente moderno: elementi di novità e ricerche in corso*, edited by Anna Maria Reggiani, 84–9. Milan: Electa.

Manderscheid, Hubertus. 2004. *Ancient Baths and Bathing: A Bibliography for the Years 1988–2001*. Portsmouth, RI: JRA.

Manderscheid, Hubertus. 2010. "*Sub nomine Caesaris quinariae*: La gestione idrica e l'architettura dell'acqua a Villa Adriana." In *Villa Adriana: Una storia mai finita: Novità e prospettive della ricerca*, edited by Marina S. Ragni, 26–33. Milan: Electa.

Martini, Wolfram. 2016. "Nymphäum und Tor: Zur Wasserkultur in Perge in Pamphylien." In *Turm und Tor: Siedlungsstrukturen in Lykien und benachbarten Kulturlandschaften*, edited by Barbara Beck-Brandt, Sabine Landstätter, and Banu Yener-Marksteiner, 279–89. Vienna: Österreichiches Archäeologisches Institut.

Mas-Guindal Lafarga, Antonio. 1992. *Los métodos informáticos en el diagnóstico de edificios antiguos: El acueducto de Segovia*. Madrid: Ministerio de Cultura.

Masi Doria, Carla, and Cosimo Cascione. 2010. "*Cura riparum*." In Riparia *dans l'empire romain: pour la définition du concept*, edited by Ella Hermon, 283–94. British Archaeological Reports-International Series 2066. Oxford: British Archaeological Reports.

Mathur, Anuradha, and Dilip da Cunha, eds. 2014. *Design in the Terrain of Water*. Philadelphia: Applied Research + Design Publishing.

Matthews, John. 2012. "The *Notitia Urbis Constantinopolitanae*." In *Two Romes: Rome and Constantinople in Late Antiquity*, edited by Lucy Grig and Gavin Kelly, 81–115. Oxford: Oxford University Press.

Mattingly, David. 2004. "Being Roman: Expressing Identity in a Provincial Setting." *JRA* 17.1: 5–25.

Mazzarino, Antonio. 1969–1970. "Un testo antico sull'inquinamento." *Helikon* 9–10: 643–45.

McInerney, Jeremy, and Ineke Sluiter. 2016a. "General Introduction." In *Valuing Landscape in Classical Antiquity: Natural Environment and Cultural Imagination*, edited by J. McInerney and I. Sluiter, 1–21. *Mnemosyne* Suppl. 393. Leiden: Brill.

McInerney, Jeremy, and Ineke Sluiter, eds. 2016b. *Valuing Landscape in Classical Antiquity: Natural Environment and Cultural Imagination*. *Mnemosyne* Suppl. 393. Leiden: Brill.

Meschini, S. 1963. "Ninfei e fontane." *Enciclopedia dell'Arte Antica, Classica, e Orientale* 5: 505–12.

Meuret, Christophe. 1996. "Le règlement de *Lamasba*: Des tables de conversion appliqués à l'irrigation." *AntAfr* 32: 87–112.

Meyers, Gretchen E. 2009. "The Divine River: Ancient Roman Identity and the Image of Tiberinus." In *The Nature and Function of Water, Baths, Bathing, and Hygiene from Antiquity through the Renaissance*, edited by Cynthia Kosso and Anne Scott, 233–47. Technology and Change in History 11. Leiden: Brill.

Miliaresis, Ismini. 2013. "Heating and Fuel Consumption in the Terme del Foro at Ostia." Ph.D. diss., University of Virginia.

Moore, Charles W. 1994. *Water and Architecture*. New York: Harry N. Abrams, Inc.

Neuerburg, Norman. 1965. *L'architettura delle fontane e dei ninfei nell'Italia antica*. Naples: Gaetano Macchiaroli Editore.

Neudecker, Richard. 1994. *Die Pracht der Latrine: zum Wandel der öffentlichen Bedürfnisanstalten in der kaiserzeitlichen Stadt*. Munich: Verlag Dr. Friedrich Pfeil.

Nieberle, Matthias. 2016. "The Archaeological Park of Baiae: New Hydrological Findings and Considerations." In *De aquaeductu atque aqua urbium Lyciae Pamphyliae Pisidiae: The Legacy of Sextus Julius Frontinus*, edited by Gilbert Wiplinger, 203–14. *BABesch* Suppl. 27. Leuven: Peeters.

Ng, Diana Y. 2007. "Manipulation of Memory: Public Buildings and Decorative Programs in Roman Cities of Asia Minor." Ph.D. diss., University of Michigan.

Nriagu, Jerome O. 1983. "Saturine Gout Among Roman Aristocrats. Did Lead Poisoning Contribute to the Fall of the Empire?" *New England Journal of Medicine* 308: 660–63.

Oestigaard, Terge. 2011. "Water." In *The Archaeology of Ritual and Religion*, edited by Timothy Insoll, 38–50. Oxford: Oxford University Press.

Oetelaar, Taylor. 2013. "Reconstructing the Baths of Caracalla." *Digital Applications in Archaeology and Cultural Heritage*. [http://dx.doi.org/10.1016/j.daach.2013.12.002].

Ohlig, Christoph P.J. 1995. "Vitruvs 'castellum aquae' und die Wasserversorgung im antiken Pompeji." *Schriftenreihe der Frontinus-Gesellschaft* 19: 124–47.

Ohlig, Christoph P.J. 2001. *De aquis Pompeiorum. Das Castellum Aquae in Pompeji: Herkunft, Zuleitung und Verteilung des Wassers*. Cicumvesuviana 4. Nijmegen: Books on Demand Nordestedt.

Ohlig, Christoph P.J. 2012. "Klimaorientierte Wassermutzung bei Hitze und Frost am Beispiel Pompejis und der Colonia Ulpia Traiana (Xanten)." In *Wasserwirtschaftliche*

Innovationen im archäologischen Kontext: Von den prähistorischen Anfängen bis zu den Metropolen der Antiken, edited by Florian Klimscha et al., 287–308. Rahden: Verlag Marie Leidorf.

Oleson, John Peter. 1984. *Greek and Roman Mechanical Water-Lifting Devices: The History of a Technology*. Toronto: University of Toronto Press.

Oleson, John Peter. 2000a. "Irrigation." In *Handbook of Ancient Water Technology*, edited by Örjan Wikander, 183–216. Technology and Change in History 2. Leiden: Brill.

Oleson, John Peter. 2000b. "Water-Lifting." In *Handbook of Ancient Water Technology*, edited by Örjan Wikander, 217–302. Technology and Change in History 2. Leiden: Brill.

Osanna, Massimo. 2015. "Zwischen Quellen und Gebirgsbächen: Wasser in Lukanischen Heiligtümern." In *Natur—Kult—Raum: Aken des internationalen Kolloquiums, Paris-Lodron-Universität Salzburg, 20–22 Jänner 2012*, edited by Katya Sporn, Sabine Ladstätter, and Michael Kerschner, 267–378. Wien: Österreichisches Archäologisches Institut.

Ostrom, Elinor. 1990. *Governing the Commons: The Evolution of Institutions for Collective Action*. Cambridge: Cambridge University Press.

Pandolfi, G. 2008. "Roma e la cultura dell'acqua: Un legame inscindibile." *Bollettino della Società geografica italiana* 13.1: 95–124.

Paniagua, David. 2016. *Sexto Julio Frontino. De aquaeductu urbis Romae/Las canalizaciones de agua de la ciudad de Roma. Estudio introductorio, traducción y notas.* Zaragoza: Libros Pórtico.

Peachin, Michael. 2004. *Frontinus and the* curae *of the* curator aquarum. Stuttgart: Franz Steiner Verlag.

Peréx, María J., and Carme Miró. 2011. "*VBI AQUAE IBI SALVS*. Atlas de aguas mineromedicinales, termas curativas y culto a las aguas en la Hispania antigua." In *Aquae Sacrae: Agua y sacralidad en la Antigüedad*, edited by Ana Costa Solé et al., 59–67. Girona: Institut de Recerca Històrica de la Universitat de Girona.

Peréx, María J., and Jesús Rodríguez Morales. 2011. "Las *stationes* con *Aquae* ... en la *Tabula* de Peutinger." *Espacio, Tiempo y Forma* 4: 153–70.

Pickett, Jordan. 2015. "Water after Antiquity in the Eastern Mediterranean: the Afterlives of Roman Hydraulic Infrastructure (300–800 CE)." PhD diss., University of Pennsylvania.

Pinto, John A. 1986. *The Trevi Fountain*. New Haven: Yale University Press.

Piranomonte, Marina, ed. 2012. *Le Terme di Caracalla*. Milan: Electa.

Piras, Susanna A.G. 2000. "Water Luxury in Roman Times: Simply a Matter of Excellent Planning and Engineering or of Politics and Philanthropy?" In *Cura Aquarum in Sicilia*, edited by Gemma C.M. Jansen, 247–53. *BABesch* Suppl. 6. Leiden: Peeters.

Piras, Susanna A.G. 2006. "Façade Nymphaea in Asia Minor: Aspendos, an Example of Massive Urban Water Imprint." In *Cura Aquarum in Ephesus*, vol. 2, edited by Gilbert Wiplinger, 397–400. *BABesch* Suppl. 12. Leuven: Peeters.

Pitts, Martin, and Miguel John Versluys, eds. 2015. *Globalization and the Roman World: World History, Connectivity and Material Culture*. Cambridge: Cambridge University Press.

Poccetti, Paolo. 1996. "Culti delle acque e stadi della vita muliebre: Dottrine misteriche e fondo religioso italic nella Tavola Osca di Agnone." In *La Tavola di Agnone nel contesto italico*, edited by Loretta Del Tutto Palma, 219–41. Florence: Leo. S. Olschki Editore.

Pont, Anne-Valérie. 2010. *Orner la cité: Enjeux culturels et politiques du paysage urbain dans l'Asie gréco-romaine*. Paris: Diffusion De Boccard.

Prayon, Friedhelm. 1990. "Wasserkulte in Etrurien." In *Der Welt der Etrusker*, edited by Huberta Heres and Max Kunze, 77–79. Berlin: Akademie-Verlag.

Purcell, Nicholas. 1995. "The Roman *Villa* and the Landscape of Production." In *Urban Society in Roman Italy*, edited by Tim J. Cornell and Kathyrn Thomas, 151–179. London: University College London.

Purcell, Nicholas. 1996. "Rome and the Management of Water: Environment, Culture, and Power." In *Human Landscapes in Classical Antiquity*, edited by Graham Shipley and John Salmon, 189–212. London: Routledge.

Purcell, Nicholas. 2012. "Rivers and the Geography of Power." *Pallas* 90: 373–87.

Rawson, Elizabeth. 1987. "*Discrimina Ordinum*: The *Lex Julia Theatralis*." *PBSR* 55: 83–114.

Reimers, Pontus. 1989. "'Opus Omnium Dictu Maximum': Literary Sources for the Knowledge of Roman City Drainage." *ORom* 17: 137–41.

Reimers, Pontus. 1991. "Roman Sewers and Sewerage Networks: Neglected Areas of Study." In *Munuscula Romana*, edited by Anne-Marie L. Touati, Eva Rystedt, and Örjan Wikander, 111–17. Stockholm: Paul Åstroms.

Remolà Vallverdú, Josep Anton, ed. 2011. *La gestión de los residuos urbanos en Hispania: Xavier Dupré Raventós (1956–2006) in Memoriam*. Madrid: Consejo Superior de Investigaciones Científicas.

Revell, Louise. 2009. *Roman Imperialism and Local Identities*. Cambridge: Cambridge University Press.

Revell, Louise. 2016. *Ways of Being Roman: Discourses of Identity in the Roman West*. Oxford: Oxbow.

Ricciardi, Maria A., and Valnea Santa Maria Scrinari. 1996. *La civilità dell'acqua in Ostia Antica*, vol. 2. Rome: Fratelli Palombi Editori.

Richard, Julian. 2007. "Roman Monumental Fountains in the Levant: Water Supply vs. Urban Aesthetics?" In *Cura Aquarum in Jordanien*, edited by Christoph Ohlig, 263–84. Schriften der DWhG Band 12. Norderstedt: DWhG.

Richard, Julian. 2012. *Water for the City, Fountains for the People: Monumental Fountains in the Roman East, An Archaeological Study of Water Management*. Turnhout: Brepols.

Richard, Julian. 2016a. "Stagnant Beauties? Some Reflections on the Speed of the Water Flow in Roman Nymphaea." In *De aquaeductu atque aqua urbium Lyciae Pamphyliae*

Pisidiae: The Legacy of Sextus Julius Frontinus, edited by Gilbert Wiplinger, 275–81. *BABesch* Suppl. 27. Leuven: Peeters.

Richard, Julian. 2016b. "Where Do We Go Now? The Archaeology of Monumental Fountains in the Roman and Early Byzantine East." In *Fountains and Water Culture in Byzantium*, edited by Brooke Shilling and Paul Stephenson, 15–35. Cambridge: Cambridge University Press.

Riera, Italo. 1994. "Le testimonianze archeologiche." In Utilitas necessaria: *Sistemi idraulici nell'Italia romana*, edited by I. Riera, 163–466. Milan: Grafiche Falletti.

Rinne, Katherine W. 1999. "The Secret Life of Roman Fountains." *Places* 12.2: 76–81.

Rinne, Katherine W. 2010. *The Waters of Rome: Aqueducts, Fountains, and the Birth of the Baroque City*. New Haven: Yale University Press.

Rinne, Katherine W. 2016. Aqua Urbis Romae: *The Waters of the City of Rome*. [www3.iath.virginia.edu/waters/]. (Last accessed 13 September 2017)

Rippon, Stephen. 2014. "Considering 'Urban Waterscapes' in Britain." *JRA* 27.2: 739–40.

Ritti, Tullia, Klaus Grewe, and Paul Kessener. 2007. "A Relief of a Water-Powered Stone Saw Mill on a Sarcophagus at Hierapolis and its Implications." *JRA* 20: 138–63.

Robert, Louis. 1977. "La titulature de Nicée et de Nicomédie: la gloire et la haine." *HSPh* 81: 211–49.

Robinson, Betsey A. 2001. "Fountains and the Culture of Water at Roman Corinth." Ph.D. diss., University of Pennsylvania.

Robinson, Betsey A. 2005. "Fountains and the Formation of Cultural Identity at Roman Corinth." In *Urban Religion in Roman Corinth: Interdisciplinary Approaches*, edited by Daniel N. Schowalter and Steven J. Friesen, 111–40. Harvard Theolological Studies 53. Cambridge, MA: Harvard University Press.

Robinson, Betsey A. 2011. *Histories of Peirene: A Corinthian Fountain in Three Millennia*. Ancient Art and Architecture in Context 2. Princeton: American School of Classical Studies at Athens.

Robinson, Betsey A. 2013. "Playing in the Sun: Hydraulic Architecture and Water Displays in Imperial Corinth." *Hesperia* 82.2: 341–84.

Robinson, Betsey A. 2016. "Landscape and Setting." In *A Companion to Greek Architecture*, edited by Margaret M. Miles, 3–14. Chichester: Wiley Blackwell.

Rodgers, Robert H. 2004. *Frontinus* De Aquaeductu Urbis Romae, *edited with an Introduction and Commentary*. Cambridge: Cambridge University Press.

Rogers, Adam C. 2013. *Water and Roman Urbanism: Towns, Waterscapes, Land Transformation and Experience in Roman Britain*. *Mnemosyne* Suppl. 355. Leiden: Brill.

Rogers, Dylan Kelby. 2013. "Il piacere d'acqua: I ninfei di Pompei." In *Ricerche a confronto: Dialoghi di antichità classiche e del vicino oriente*, edited by Viola Gheller, 154–69. Il Tempo nel Tempo 6. Montorso Vicentino: Edizioni Saecula.

Rogers, Dylan Kelby. 2015. "Water-Display and Meaning in the High Roman Empire." Ph.D. diss., University of Virginia.

Rogers, Dylan Kelby. 2016. Review of *The Archaeology of Sanitation in Roman Italy: Toilets, Sewers, and Water Systems*, by A.O. Koloski-Ostrow. *CJ Online* 2016.03.01. [https://cj.camws.org/sites/default/files/reviews/2016.03.01%20Rogers%20on%20Koloski-Ostrow.pdf]. (Last accessed 13 September 2017)

Rogers, Dylan Kelby. 2018. "Shifting Tides: Approaches to the Public Water-Displays of Roman Greece." In *Great Waterworks of Roman Greece: Aqueducts and Monumental Fountains, Function in Context*, edited by Georgia Aristodemou and Theodosios P. Tassios, 173–92. Oxford: Archeopress.

Rogers, Dylan Kelby. Forthcoming. "Water-Displays in Roman Greece: A Sensorial Approach."

Rowland, Ingrid D., and Thomas Noble Howe. 1999. *Vitruvius: Ten Books on Architecture*. Cambridge: Cambridge University Press.

Rubinstein, Lene. 1995. "Pausanias as a Source for the Classical Greek *Polis*." In *Studies in the Ancient Greek* Polis, edited by Mogens H. Hansen and Kurt Raaflaub, 211–19. Stuttgart: Franz Steiner Verlag.

Saastamoinen, Ari. 2003. "The Literary Character of Frontinus' *De aquaeductu*." In *Technology, Ideology, Water: From Frontinus to the Renaissance and Beyond*, edited by Christer Bruun and A. Saastamoinen, 15–39. Rome: Institutum Romanum Finlandiae.

Sabri, Raghid, Broder Merkel, and Marion Tichomirowa. 2016. "Watermill as Sustainable Development." In *De aquaeductu atque aqua urbium Lyciae Pamphyliae Pisidiae: The Legacy of Sextus Julius Frontinus*, edited by Gilbert Wiplinger, 313–20. *BABesch* Suppl. 27. Leuven: Peeters.

Saller, Richard. 2002. "Framing the Debate over Growth in the Ancient Economy." In *The Ancient Economy*, edited by Walter Scheidel and Sitta von Reden, 251–69. Oxford: Oxford University Press.

Salowey, Christina A. 1994. "Herakles and the Waterworks in the Peloponnesos: Mycenean Dams, Classical Fountains, and Roman Aqueducts." In *Archaeology in the Peloponnese: New Excavations and Research*, edited by Kenneth Sheedy, 77–94. Oxford: Oxbow.

Salza Prina Ricotti, Eugenia. 1998. "Adriano: Architettura del verde e dell'acqua." In *Horti Romani*, edited by Maddalena Cima and Eugenio La Rocca, 363–400. Rome: "L'Erma" di Bretschneider.

Scarborough, John. 1984. "The Myth of Lead Poisoning Among the Romans: An Essay Review." *Journal of the History of Medicine* 39: 469–75.

Schama, Simon. 1995. *Landscape and Memory*. New York: Alfred Knopf.

Scheid, John. 1991. "Sanctuaries et thermes sous l'empire." *Les thermes Romains*, [no ed.], 205–14. Collection de l'École Française de Rome 142. Rome: École Française de Rome.

Scheid, John. 1996. "Pline le Jeune et les sanctuaires d'Italie. Observations sur le *Lettres* IV, 1, VIII, 8 et IX, 39." In Splendidissima civitas*: Études d'histoire romaine en homage* *à François Jacques*, edited by André Chastagnol, Ségolène Demougin, and Claude Lepelley, 241–58. Paris: Publications de la Sorbonne.

Schmitz, Dirk, and Maike Sieler, eds. 2013. *Überall zu Hause und doch fremd: Römer unterwegs*. Petersburg: Imhof.

Schmölder-Veit, Andrea. 2009. *Brunnen in den Städten des westlichen Römischen Reichs*. Palilia 19. Wiesbaden: Dr. Ludwig Reichert Verlag.

Scobie, Alex. 1986. "Slums, Sanitation, and Mortality in the Roman World." *Klio* 68: 399–433.

Sear, Frank B. 2006. *Roman Theaters: An Architectural Study*. Oxford: Oxford University Press.

Segal, Arthur. 1997. *From Function to Monument: Urban Landscapes of Roman Palestine, Syria, and Provincia Arabia*. Oxbow Monograph 66. Oxford: Oxbow.

Seigne, Jacques. 2006. "Water-Powered Stone Saws in Late Antiquity: First Step on the Way to Industrialisation?" In *Cura Aquarum in Ephesus*, vol. 2, edited by Gilbert Wiplinger, 371–78. *BABesch* Suppl. 12. Leuven: Peeters.

Seppilli, Anita. 1977. *Sacralità dell'acqua e sacrilegio dei ponti: Persistenza di simboli e dinamica culturale*. Palermo: Sellerio Editore.

Settis, Salvatore. 1973. "'Esedra' e 'Ninfeo' nella terminologia architettonica del mondo romano: Dell'età repubblicana alla tarda antichità." *ANRW* 1.4: 661–745.

Shaw, Brent D. 1982. "Lamasba: An Ancient Irrigation Community." *AntAfr* 18: 61–103.

Shaw, Brent D. 1991. "The Noblest Monuments and the Smallest Things: Wells, Walls, and Aqueducts in the Making of Roman Africa." In *Future Currents in Aqueduct Studies*, edited by A. Trevor Hodge, 63–92. Leeds: Francis Cairns.

Shipley, Graham, and John Salmon, eds. 1996. *Human Landscapes in Classical Antiquity: Environment and Culture*. London: Routledge.

Sodini, Jean-Pierre, Tony Kozelj, and Manuela Wurch-Koželj. 2016. *Le nymphée d'une maison de l'Antiquité Tardive à Thasos (terrains Tokatlis/Divanakis/Voulgaridis)*. Études Thasiennes 24. Athens: École Française d'Athènes.

Spawforth, Antony J.S. 2012. *Greece and the Augustan Cultural Revolution*. Cambridge: Cambridge University Press.

Spencer, Diana. 2007. "Rome at a Gallop: Livy on Not Gazing, Jumping, or Toppling into the Void." In *The Sites of Rome: Time, Space, and Memory*, edited by David H.J. Lamour and D. Spencer, 66–83. Oxford: Oxford University Press.

Spencer, Diana. 2010. *Roman Landscape: Culture and Identity*. *G&R*: New Surveys in the Classics 39. Cambridge: Cambridge University Press.

Stähli, Adrian. 2013. "Women Bathing: Displaying Female Attractiveness on Greek Vases." In *Greek Baths and Bathing Culture: New Discoveries and Approaches*, edited by Sandra K. Lucore and Monika Trümper, 11–21. *BABesch* Suppl. 23. Leuven: Peeters.

Stein, Richard J.B. 2014. *The Roman Water Pump: Unique Evidence for Roman Mastery of Mechanical Engineering*. Montagnac: M. Mergoil.

Stephenson, Paul. 2016. "The Serpent Column Fountain." In *Fountains and Water Culture in Byzantium*, edited by Brooke Shilling and P. Stephenson, 87–102. Cambridge: Cambridge University Press.

Stephenson, Paul, and Ragnar Hedlund. 2016. "Monumental Waterworks in Late Antique Constantinople." In *Fountains and Water Culture in Byzantium*, edited by Brooke Shilling and P. Stephenson, 15–35. Cambridge: Cambridge University Press.

Strang, Veronica. 2004. *The Meaning of Water*. Oxford: Berg.

Strang, Veronica. 2005. "Common Senses: Water, Sensory Experience, and the Generation of Meaning." *Journal of Material Culture* 10.1: 92–120.

Strang, Veronica. 2006. "Introduction: Fluidscapes: Water, Identity, and the Senses." *Worldview* 10.2: 147–54.

Strang, Veronica. 2008. "The Social Construction of Water." In *Handbook of Landscape Archaeology*, edited by Bruno David and Julian Thomas, 123–30. Walnut Creek, CA: Left Coast Press.

Strang, Veronica. 2012. "Extremely Private: Water Trading and the Commoditization of Water." In *Water, Cultural Diversity and Global Environmental Change: Emerging Trends, Sustainable Futures?*, edited by Barbara R. Johnston et al., 257–60. Paris: UNESCO.

Symmes, Marilyn, ed. 1998. *Fountains: Splash and Spectacle, Water and Design from the Renaissance to the Present.* New York: Rizzoli.

Taback, Natalie. 2002. "Untangling the Muses: A Comprehensive Study of Sculptures of Muses in the Greek and Roman World." Ph.D. diss., Harvard University.

Taylor, Rabun. 2000. *Public Needs and Private Pleasures: Water Distribution, the Tiber River, and the Urban Development of Ancient Rome*. Studia Archaeologica 109. Rome: "L'Erma" di Bretschneider.

Taylor, Rabun. 2009. "River Raptures: Containment and Control of Water in Greek and Roman Constructions of Identity." In *The Nature and Function of Water, Baths, Bathing, and Hygiene from Antiquity through the Renaissance*, edited by Cynthia Kosso and Anne Scott, 21–42. Technology and Change in History 11. Leiden: Brill.

Taylor, Rabun. 2010. "Bread and Water. Septimius Severus and the *Curator Aquarum et Minuciae*." *MAAR* 55: 199–220.

Taylor, Rabun, Katherine W. Rinne, Edward O'Neill, and Michael O'Neill. 2010. "A Grotto-Shrine at the Headwaters of the Aqua Traiana." *JRA* 23: 358–75.

Taylor, Rabun, Giovanni Isidori, Edward O'Neill, Michael O'Neill, and Katherine W. Rinne. 2016. "New Wine for Old Bottles: New Research on the Sources of the Aqua Traiana." *Waters of Rome* 4. [www3.iath.virginia.edu/waters/Journal9Taylor_et_al.pdf]. (Last accessed 13 September 2017)

Thébert, Yvon. 2003. *Thermes romains d'Afrique du nord et leur context méditerranéen*. Rome: École Française de Rome.

Thomas, Edmund. 2007. *Monumentality and the Roman Empire: Architecture in the Antonine Age*. Oxford: Oxford University Press.

Thomas, Edmund. 2012. "Water and the Display of Power in Augustan Rome: The So-Called 'Villa Claudia' at Anguillara Sabazia." *Water History* 4.1: 57–78.

Thomas, Julian. 2006. "Archaeologies of Place and Landscape." In *Archaeological Theory Today*, edited by Ian Hodder, 165–86. London: Blackwell.

Thomas, Robert, and Andrew I. Wilson. 1994. "Water Supply for Roman Farms in Latium and South Etruria." *PBSR* 62: 139–96.

Thüry, Günther E. 2001. *Müll und Marmorsäulen: Siedlungshygiene in der römischen Antike*. Mainz am Rhein: Verlag Philipp von Zabern.

Tölle-Kastenbein, Renate. 1990. *Antike Wasserkultur*. Munich: Verlag C.H. Beck.

Tölle-Kastenbein, Renate. 1994. *Das archaische Wasserleitungsnetz für Athen und seine späteren Bauphasen*. Mainz am Rhein: Verlag Philipp von Zabern.

Tomasello, Francesco. 2005. *Fontane e ninfei minori di Leptis Magna*. Monografie di Archeologia Libica 27. Rome: "L'Erma" di Bretschneider.

Toner, Jerry, ed. 2014. *A Cultural History of the Senses in Antiquity*. London: Bloomsbury.

Topták, Tomáš. 2009. "Die Symbolik des Wassers." *Anodos* 9: 95–106.

Traversari, Gustavo. 1960. *Gli spettacoli in acqua nel teatro tardo-antico*. Rome: "L'Erma" di Bretschneider.

Trümper, Monika. 2013. "Introduction." In *Greek Baths and Bathing Culture: New Discoveries and Approaches*, edited by Sandra K. Lucore and M. Trümper, 1–10. *BABesch* Suppl. 23. Leuven: Peeters.

Tsiolis, Vassilis. 2013. "The Baths at Fregellae and the Transition from *Balneion* to *Balneum*." In *Greek Baths and Bathing Culture: New Discoveries and Approaches*, edited by Sandra K. Lucore and Monika Trümper, 89–111. *BABesch* Suppl. 23. Leuven: Peeters.

Ucko, Peter J., and Robert Layton. 1999a. "Introduction: Gazing on the Landscape and Encountering the Environment." In *The Archaeology and Anthropology of Landscape: Shaping Your Landscape*, edited by P.J. Ucko and R. Layton, 1–20. London: Routledge.

Ucko, Peter J., and Robert Layton, eds. 1999b. *The Archaeology and Anthropology of Landscape: Shaping Your Landscape*. London: Routledge.

Uğurlu, Nur Banu. 2009. *The Roman Nymphaea in the Cities of Asia Minor: Function in Context*. Saarbrücken: VDM Verlag.

Uytterhoeven, Inge. 2012. "Private Bathing in Imperial and Late Antique Asia Minor: A Contribution to the Study of Ancient Bathing from a Private Point of View." In *SPA, Sanitas per Aquam: Proceedings of the International Frontinus-Symposium on the Technical and Cultural History of Ancient Baths*, edited by Ralf Kreiner and Wolfram Letzner, 289–93. *BABesch* Suppl. 21. Leuven: Peeters.

Van Deman, Esther B. 1934. *The Building of the Roman Aqueducts*. Washington: Carnegie Institution of Washington.

Van Oyen, Astrid. 2015. "Globalisation and Material Culture: The Road Ahead." *JRA* 28.2: 640–51.

Vitti, Paolo. 2016. *Building Roman Greece: Innovation in Vaulted Construction in the Peloponnese*. Studia Archeologia 206. Rome: "L'Erma" di Bretschneider.

Von Falkenstein-Wirth, Vera. 2011. *Das Quellheiligtum von Vicarello (Aquae Apollinares): Ein Kultort von der Bronzezeit bis zum Ende des Kaiserreichs*. Mainz: Verlag Philipp von Zabern.

Walker, Susan. 1979. "The Architectural Development of Roman Nymphaea in Greece." D.Phil. thesis, University of London.

Walker, Susan. 1987. "Roman Nymphaea in the Greek World." In *Roman Architecture in the Greek World*, edited by Sarah Macready and F.H. Thompson, 60–71. London: Thames and Hudson.

Wallace-Hadrill, Andrew. 2008. *Rome's Cultural Revolution*. Cambridge: Cambridge University Press.

Ward-Perkins, Brian. 2012. "Old and New Rome Compared: The Rise of Constantinople." In *Two Romes: Rome and Constantinople in Late Antiquity*, edited by Lucy Grig and Gavin Kelly, 53–80. Oxford: Oxford University Press.

Wassenhoven, Maria-Evdokia. 2012. *The Bath in Greece in Classical Antiquity: The Peloponnese*. British Archaeological Reports-International Series 2368. Oxford: British Archaeological Reports.

Wasserversorgung II. 1987. *Die Wasserversorgung antiker Städte. Pergamon. Recht/Verwaltung. Brunnen/Nymphäen. Bauelemente. Geschichte der Wasserversorgung* 2. Mainz am Rhein: Verlag Philipp von Zabern.

Wasserversorgung II. 2013. *Die Wasserversorgung im antiken Rom Sextus Iulius Frontinus, sein Werk in lateinisch und Deutsch und begleitende Fachaufsätze*. München: DIV Deutscher Industrieverlag.

Wasserversorgung III. 1988. *Die Wasserversorgung antiker Städte. Mensch und Wasser. Mitteleuropa. Thermen. Bau/Materialen. Hygiene. Geschichte der Wasserversorgung* 3. Mainz am Rhein: Verlag Philipp von Zabern.

Weiss, Cecelia F. 2011. "Living Fluidly: Uses and Meanings of Water in Asia Minor (Second Century BCE–Second Century CE)." Ph.D. diss., Brown University.

Welch, Katherine E. 2007. *The Roman Amphitheater: From its Origins to the Colosseum*. Cambridge: Cambridge University Press.

Wellbrock, Kai, ed. 2017. *Cura Aquarum in Greece: Proceedings of the 16th International Conference on the History of Water Management and Hydraulic Engineering in the Mediterranean Region, Athens, Greece, 28–30 March 2015*. Schriften der DWhG Band 27. Sieburg: DWhG.

Wescoat, James L. 2013. "Water and Waterworks in Garden Archaeology." In *Sourcebook for Garden Archaeology*, edited by Amina-Aïcha Malek, 421–51. Bern: Peter Lang.

Wikander, Örjan. 2000. "The Water-Mill." In *Handbook of Ancient Water Technology*, edited by Ö. Wikander, 371–400. Technology and Change in History 2. Leiden: Brill.

Wiles, David. 2003. *A Short History of Western Performance Space.* Cambridge: Cambridge University Press.

Williams, Gareth D. 2012. *The Cosmic Viewpoint: A Study of Seneca's* Natural Questions. Oxford: Oxford University Press.

Wilson, Andrew I. 1995. "Running Water and Social Status in North Africa." In *North Africa from Antiquity to Islam*, edited by Mark Horton and Thomas E.J. Weidemann, 52–6. Bristol: Centre for Mediterranean Studies (University of Bristol).

Wilson, Andrew I. 1998. "Water Supply in Ancient Carthage." In *Carthage Papers: The Early Colony's Economy, Water Supply, a Private Bath, and the Mobilization of State Olive Oil*, edited by John T. Peña, 65–102. *JRA* Suppl. 28. Portsmouth, RI: JRA.

Wilson, Andrew I. 1999. "Deliveries *extra urbem*: Aqueducts and the Countryside." *JRA* 12: 314–29.

Wilson, Andrew I. 2000a. "Drainage and Sanitation." In *Handbook of Ancient Water Technology*, edited by Örjan Wikander, 151–79. Technology and Change in History 2. Leiden: Brill.

Wilson, Andrew I. 2000b. "The Aqueducts of Italy and Gaul." *JRA* 13.1: 597–604.

Wilson, Andrew I. 2000c. "The Water-Mills on the Janiculum." *MAAR* 45: 219–46.

Wilson, Andrew I. 2001. "Urban Water Storage, Distribution, and Usage." In *Water Use and Hydraulics in the Roman City*, edited by Ann Olga Koloski-Ostrow, 83–95. Dubuque, IA: Kendall/Hunt Publishing.

Wilson, Andrew I. 2002. "Machines, Power and the Ancient Economy." *JRS* 92: 1–32.

Wilson, Andrew I. 2006. "The Economic Impact of Technological Advances in the Roman Construction Industry." In *Innovazione tecnica e progresso economico nel mondo romano*, edited by Elio Lo Casio, 225–36. Bari: Edipuglia.

Wilson, Andrew I. 2008. "Hydraulic Engineering and Water Supply." In *The Oxford Handbook of Engineering and Technology in the Classical World*, edited by John Peter Oleson, 285–318. Oxford: Oxford University Press.

Wilson, Andrew I. 2009. "Foggaras in Ancient North Africa or How to Marry a Berber Princess." In *Contrôle et distribution de l'eau dans le Maghreb antique et médiéval*, [no ed.], 19–39. Rome: École Française de Rome.

Wilson, Andrew I. 2012. "Water, Power, and Culture in the Roman and Byzantine Worlds: An Introduction." *Water History* 4.1: 1–9.

Wilson, Andrew I. 2017. "Rivers, Wadis, and Climate in North Africa: Torrents and Drought." In *Fluvial Landscapes in the Roman World*, edited by Tyler V. Franconi, 111–126. *JRA* Suppl. 104. Portsmouth, RI: JRA.

Wilson, Roger J.A. 1996. "*Tot aquarum tam multis necessariis molibus …*: Recent Studies on Aqueducts and Water Supply." *JRA* 9: 5–29.

Wiplinger, Gilbert, ed. 2011. *Historische Wasserleitungen. Gestern—Heute—Morgen: Tagungsband des Internationalen Frontinus-Symposiums. Wien, 19.–23. Oktober 2011. BABesch* Suppl. 24. Leuven: Peeters.

Wiplinger, Gilbert. 2016a. "Der hadrianische und antoninische Değirmendere Aquädukt von Ephesos: 10 Jahre nach dem Ephesos-Symposium." In *De aquaeductu atque aqua urbium Lyciae Pamphyliae Pisidiae: The Legacy of Sextus Julius Frontinus*, edited by G. Wiplinger, 55–64. *BABesch* Suppl. 27. Leuven: Peeters.

Wiplinger, Gilbert, ed. 2016b. *De aquaeductu atque aqua urbium Lyciae Pamphyliae Pisidiae: The Legacy of Sextus Julius Frontinus. BABesch* Suppl. 27. Leuven: Peeters.

Wiplinger, Gilbert, and Wolfram Letzner, eds. 2017. *Wasserwesen zur Zeit des Frontinus, Bauwerke—Technik—Kultur: Tagungsband des internationalen Frontinus-Symposiums, Trier, 25–29. Mai 2016. BABesch* Suppl. 32. Leuven: Peeters.

Wissowa, Georg. 1902. *Religion und Kultus der Römer*. Munich: C.H. Beck.

Witcher, Robert. 2006. "Broken Pots and Meaningless Dots? Surveying the Rural Landscapes of Roman Italy." *PBSR* 74: 39–72.

Wylie, John. 2007. *Landscape*. New York: Routledge.

Yegül, Fikret K. 1992. *Baths and Bathing in Classical Antiquity*. New York: The Architectural History Foundation.

Yegül, Fikret K. 1996. "The Thermo-Mineral Complex at Baiae and the *De Balneis Puteolanis*." *The Art Bulletin* 78.1: 137–62.

Yegül, Fikret K. 2010. *Bathing in the Roman World*. Cambridge: Cambridge University Press.

Yegül, Fikret K. 2013. "Thermal Matters: Intersected Legacies of Greek and Roman Baths and Bathing Culture." In *Greek Baths and Bathing Culture: New Discoveries and Approaches*, edited by Sandra K. Lucore and Monika Trümper, 73–88. *BABesch* Suppl. 23. Leuven: Peeters.

Yegül, Fikret K., and Tristan Couch. 2003. "Building a Roman Bath for the Cameras." *JRA* 16: 153–77.

Zajac, Natascha. 1999. "The *Thermae*: A Policy of Public Health or Personal Legitimization?" In *Roman Baths and Bathing: Proceedings of the First International Conference on Roman Baths held at Bath, England, 30 March–4 April 1992*, edited by Janet DeLaine and David E. Johnson, 99–105. Portsmouth, RI: JRA.

Zarmakoupi, Mantha. 2014. *Designing for Luxury on the Bay of Naples: Villas and Landscapes (c. 100 BCE–79 CE)*. Oxford: Oxford University Press.

www.ingramcontent.com/pod-product-compliance
Lightning Source LLC
Chambersburg PA
CBHW031328230926
51848CB00001B/133